ABT

ACPL ITEM
DISCARDE

3 1833 0

D0253520

STOPPING
INFLAMMATION

STOPPING
INFLAMMATION

Relieving the Cause
of Degenerative Diseases

NANCY APPLETON, PhD
with G. N. Jacobs

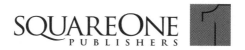

SQUAREONE
PUBLISHERS

COVER DESIGNER: Phaedra Mastrocola
EDITOR: Larry Trivieri, Jr.
TYPESETTERS: Gary A. Rosenberg and Terry Wiscovitch

The information and advice contained in this book are based upon the research and the personal and professional experiences of the author. They are not intended as a substitute for consulting with a health care professional. The publisher and author are not responsible for any adverse effects or consequences resulting from the use of any of the suggestions, preparations, or procedures discussed in this book. All matters pertaining to your physical health should be supervised by a health care professional. It is a sign of wisdom, not cowardice, to seek a second or third opinion.

Square One Publishers
115 Herricks Road
Garden City Park, NY 11040
(516) 535-2010 • (877) 900-BOOK
www.squareonepublishers.com

Library of Congress Cataloging-in-Publication Data

Appleton, Nancy.
    Stopping inflammation : relieving the cause of degenerative diseases / Nancy Appleton with G.N. Jacobs.
        p. cm.
    Includes bibliographical references and index.
    ISBN 0-7570-0148-3 (pbk.)
    1. Inflammation—Popular works. 2. Chronic diseases—Etiology—Popular works. I. Jacobs, G. N. II. Title.
RB131.A675   2005
616'.0473—dc22

                                                        2004014335

Copyright © 2005 by Nancy Appleton

All rights reserved. No part of this publication may be reproduced, stored in a retrieval system, or transmitted, in any form or by any means, electronic, mechanical, photocopying, recording, or otherwise, without the prior written permission of the publisher.

Printed in the United States of America

10   9   8   7   6   5   4   3   2   1

Contents

PART THREE

Guidelines for Preventing and Reversing Inflammation

Acknowledgments

I would like to acknowledge the life's work of the many pioneering scientists and nutritionists who have enabled me to find my own course in the search for truth. They have provided the light in an otherwise darkened path. In regard to this book, I would like to thank Greg N. Jacobs for all his work and effort in making this volume what it is. Add to that a word of praise for Mihir Upadhyaya who needs to be recognized and thanked for reviewing my manuscript for correct medical information and better organization. Special thanks go to my children who have put up with my ideas in nutrition for so many years. In spite of me or because of me, they are the picture of health.

A special thanks goes to Dr. Carolyn Dean, a medical doctor and naturopathic doctor, who wrote Chapter 8 of this book. Because of her training in both disciplines, she is able to effectively bridge the gap between allopathic and alternative medicine. She has written several books on health and wellness. *Natural Prescriptions for Common Ailments* is a useful health encyclopedia and *The Miracle of Magnesium* is her most recent book. Currently, Dr. Dean is an advisor to www.yeastconnection.com and www.curesnaturally.com. Along with Delia Quigley, Dr. Dean runs Body Rejuvenation Cleanse classes in Manhattan, New Jersey, and by teleconference to help detoxify people in an increasingly toxic world. You can visit Dr. Dean's website at www.carolyndean.com or at www.brcleanse.com.

Most of all, I dedicate this book to anyone who has not found answers to his or her health problems. I hope this book helps.

—N.A.

Introduction

Degenerative diseases appear to be caused or complicated by a process few medical researchers suspected until quite recently: *inflammation*. Scientists have long linked edema, arthritis, and inflammatory bowel disease to inflammation, but have only recently implicated the process to diabetes, certain cancers, and other unsolvable degenerative conditions. The latest research links heart disease more to various inflammatory conditions (those ending with 'itis') than to high cholesterol.[1]

Inflammation has always played a role in infections. Catch a cold or fever and the nose runs, coughing sets in, temperature rises, and all the other great symptoms that children pray for as an excuse to ditch school appear. All of these symptoms are expressions of the inflammatory process. Another form of inflammation has to do with insults to the body, such as parasites, fungi, bruises, broken bones, and smoking. Healthy immune systems use inflammation to right an unbalanced body; when the job is done, inflammation and other symptoms go away.

Blood tests often show chronic, low-grade inflammation in the body. All of the known related problems have been studied and inflammation can't be linked to any specific cause. Maybe investigators aren't looking in the right direction for answers. Where does this inflammation with no known cause come from? Is there a way that we can stop this process before it even gets started? Can we prevent diseases? Are you tired of taking anti-inflammatory pills? Are you inflicted with an acute, chronic, or degenerative disease and still searching for an answer? This book will give you a fresh look at your health and how to heal yourself.

Research has shown me that many of the serious, unsolved diseases of modern civilization are expressions of chronic inflammatory processes. Medical therapy is often directed at *controlling symptoms* rather than removing their *cause*. My intent is to show you how your own lifestyle can cause inflammation, resulting in disease. I will then provide you with techniques you can use, techniques to effectively respond to an out-of-control immune system and prevent or naturally abort the inflammation process.

Throughout this book, my objective is four-fold:

1. To present the latest research that supports the link between inflammation and disease.

2. To outline alternative causes for conditions that are presently listed in the mainstream literature as having "unknown cause."

3. To reiterate the importance of finding the sources of your health problems.

4. To show you how to change your lifestyle to remove the problem of inflammation.

At the beginning of each condition listed in Chapter 5, I have given other names, or other diseases with similar problems, for the first disease on the list. Many times these diseases are not mentioned in the chapter, but the information applies to all the diseases.

Pass with me now through to the other side of the looking glass, taking the first steps on your journey to good health. We begin with an understanding of inflammation itself, which will be covered in the next chapter.

PART ONE

Understanding Inflammation

1

Inflammation and Its Causes

WHAT IS INFLAMMATION?

Inflammation is the body's natural response to injury, infection, or a foreign invader that may cause an acute or chronic reaction. The inflammatory response serves several important functions in the body, which are listed below.

1. The body tries to defend itself against what it perceives as a foreign invader (virus, bacteria, fungi, etc.).

2. The body attempts to detoxify (See Chapter 8).

3. The body wants to facilitate healing.

Inflammation is necessary for healing, but when it becomes chronic and gets out of control, problems begin. The chronic reaction is usually a low-grade reaction. We have all experienced various symptoms related to cuts and bruises, or infectious diseases like the cold or flu. Pus running out of an infected cut is a warning sign, as are runny noses, watery eyes, and coughing. Any disease ending in 'itis' refers to an inflammatory condition, such as arthritis and bronchitis. But other diseases can also result from the inflammation process, and any cell, tissue, or organ in the body can be affected by it.

TYPES OF INFLAMMATION

Included below are definitions and examples of the types of inflammation that will be discussed throughout the book.

Acute Inflammation

Acute inflammation is the immediate defense reaction of our body tissue to injuries or foreign invaders. Symptoms can involve any or all of the following: redness, heat, swelling, pain, and/or loss of function of the affected body part. Blood cells dilate, amplifying blood flow to the affected area, resulting in a warm flush from the increased blood flow to that area.

Swelling occurs when excess fluid, infiltration of cells, and greater volume of connective tissue affects the area after blood flow is boosted. The area feels pain created by the prostaglandins (fatty acid immune mediators) and sensory nerves that are stretched during swelling. Loss of function at the site springs from damaged tissue replacement, pain, joint swelling, or scar tissue which contracts as it matures in a chronic area.

Damaged tissue is replaced when white blood cells enter and engulf bacteria and other foreign particles. Similar cells from nearby tissues remove and consume dead cells, sometimes with the production of pus, jump starting the healing process. Acute inflammation is usually short-lived and disappears within a matter of days.[1]

Chronic Inflammation

Chronic low-grade inflammation is a continual response of the immune system to a perceived ongoing problem. Healing does not occur and symptoms can be similar to the acute form but may subside to reoccur in the future. Unfortunately, inflammatory conditions can linger for years and sometimes a lifetime. The end result can be internal scarring and degenerative diseases.[2]

Sometimes a person suffering from chronic inflammation has no symptoms, nor annoying irritations. Although the person feels fine, a blood test can show chronic low-grade inflammation going on in the bloodstream or in other parts of the body. This chronic condition is most harmful because a person is not usually aware that a problem exists in his or her body. Such unseen problems are implicated in many degenerative diseases that are the primary focus of this book. More information on testing for chronic inflammation is presented in Chapter 6.

The acute inflammation can become chronic, creating a long-term problem. *Often, however, chronic inflammation occurs as a primary event, with no preceding period of acute symptoms.*

WHAT CAUSES INFLAMMATION?

Many times it is difficult to pinpoint the causes of chronic low-grade inflammation, which seems to put otherwise healthy people at risk for various diseases. Dr. Peter Libby, a professor of medicine at Harvard Medical School in Boston, says: "I think the first thing we have is an epidemic of unhealthy lifestyles, and the way in which the lifestyle is wreaking its havoc is through inflammation." Before symptoms occur, the immune system has to perceive something as a threat from one or more of the following categories:

1. Microbial infections—Viruses, bacteria, parasites, and fungi can cause the immune system to secrete various white blood cells that will cause inflammation.

2. Surgery—including general surgery, periodontal surgery, dental implants, and transplants. (See Chapter 5.)

3. Physical agents—Tissue damage may occur through physical trauma (a bruise, a broken bone), ultraviolet or other ionizing radiation, burns or excessive cooling (frostbite).

4. Vaccinations[3]—Vaccinations used for a variety of diseases; whether traveler's ailments, influenza, rabies, or other sicknesses, all can cause inflammation.

5. Chemicals—You might breathe in chemicals from household cleaners or agricultural products such as pesticides that can provoke inflammation and gross tissue damage. (See Chapter 3.)

6. High blood pressure—A great many of the population have high blood pressure and do not realize inflammation is also a problem. (See Chapter 5.)

7. Estrogen therapy—Oral estrogens increase inflammation with thrombotic (blood clotting) consequences.[4]

8. Smoking and tobacco usage are sources of inflammation.[5]

9. AGEs—Advanced glycation end products are a source of inflammation due to excessive sugar in the diet and eating overprocessed food. (See Chapter 4.)

10. Free radicals (unstable molecules with open electron ports) causing oxidative stress cause inflammation. (See Chapter 4.)

11. Obesity—The more obese, the more the inflammation. (See Chapter 5.)

12. Chronic fatigue—Chronic fatigue puts stress on the body and causes inflammation.[6]

13. Hypersensitivity reactions—Hypersensitivity, an overly powerful reaction, occurs when the immune system reacts to an otherwise non-invasive substance as a foreign invader, causing inflammation and tissue damage.[7] Allergies to common substances such as pollen, animal dander, gas fumes, or other agents, as well as reactions to food can cause hypersensitivities. (See Chapter 3.)

WHAT HAPPENS WHEN THE IMMUNE SYSTEM FALTERS?

The immune system is composed of the thymus gland, the spleen, the lymph nodes, and the bone marrow. These organs manufacture T-cells (immune system regulators made in the thymus), B-cells (white blood cells made in the bone marrow), immunoglobulins (antibodies), and complements (blood immune proteins designed to kill cells). However, these cells can be easily damaged by germs, chemicals, partially digested foods, indiscriminate use of antibiotics, and other environmental stress factors. This causes inflammation that the immune system must deal with. When inflammation is excessive, the immune system can become overwhelmed and unable to function properly.

A healthy immune system includes cells we call circulating immune complexes (CICs). CICs are made up of the foreign invader or antigen and white blood cells called antibodies. This is the normal way that the immune system removes what it perceives as a foreign invader from the body. But sometimes there are too many CICs for the immune system to deal with. When the body becomes overwhelmed with CICs, the immune system will finally give up and say "this is all I can do, I am exhausted" and stop functioning properly. Symptoms of all kinds then develop in the body, becoming the precursor to disease.

People with a weakened immune system are more susceptible to infectious and degenerative diseases, such as herpes, tonsillitis, influenza, pneumonia, skin infections, AIDS, arthritis, cancer, cardiovascular disorders, chronic fatigue, and other degenerative diseases. Universal hypersensitivities may also develop in suppressed immune systems. People with chronic fatigue and environmental illness have immune systems that become overwhelmed with CICs. These people develop allergies to many things in their environment, whether chemicals, foods, or inhalants (dust, molds and pollens). These allergies may result in reactions occurring in various organs of the body. It is possible for a person to become so allergic to a normally tolerated food that a violent reaction may result anywhere in the body.

WHAT HAPPENS IN AN INFLAMMATORY REACTION?

Inflammation results from the subsequent release of tissue hormones called histamines (hormones primarily associated with anaphylaxis, an immune reaction characterized by a drop in blood pressure, swelling, short breath, and wheezing), and kinins (inflammatory mediators related to blood vessel dilation). The picture becomes crowded with other chemicals that contribute to the process, including the prevalent and well-studied cytokines (proteins secreted by inflammatory white blood cells), and the lesser known eosinophils (leukocytes with a fondness for parasites, related to allergic reactions), prostaglandins, leukotrienes (another inflammatory substance), free radicals, serotonin (neurotransmitter), interleukin (proteins regulating immunity), and insulin (a sugar regulator). Tissues heat up and swell in an attempt to bring more blood and white blood cells to the region to scavenge the invader. Mast cells (a type of leukocyte) release histamine into the bloodstream and adjacent tissues, a process enhanced by high levels of adrenaline, calcium, and phosphorus, along with reduced magnesium levels.

Normally, CICs pass through the liver and are recycled in the body. The liver can become overwhelmed with these substances, causing disturbances in many organs. This forces other immune structures to activate, creating more problems. The immune system knows of no other way to heal the sick area.

An individual's genetic blueprint will determine where CICs may lodge. If there is a weakness somewhere in the body, the immune system will attack that location. Inflammation will move right into the unhealthy area to attempt healing. Macrophages (a class of white blood cells that hunt invaders) may act as a secondary line of defense, attacking CICs in the bloodstream or in the lungs. If CICs are not removed, they may trigger a cascade of events that lead to multiple symptoms, and sometimes tissue damage.

CICs activate complement, a circulating system of twenty-five proteins that interact to produce a variety of defensive molecular weapons. The primary purpose of complement is to act like a cellular can opener, spilling the cell's innards into the body, resulting in cellular death. In normal conditions, certain complement products are essential to clear CICs and stop the cascade of cell damage. Individuals with nutritional deficiencies are at greater risk of developing immune complexes. When activated abnormally, the complement system changes, producing powerful effects that can include anaphylaxis. Many ailments that at first glance do not seem to have much in common actually have inflammation as an underlying reason for their pathology.[8]

Each disease may trigger different white blood cells that might make the inflammatory process different, but the bottom line is that in all inflammatory processes the immune system becomes overwhelmed. Usually a swarm of lymphocytes (another class of white blood cells serving the immune system) infiltrate the inflamed tissue. Any part of the body can be involved in an immune response to a foreign invader. The normal homeostatic mechanisms become overwhelmed, losing their ability to regain and maintain homeostasis. The result is disease laying in wait like an animal ready to attack.

THE SEARCH GOES ON

The medical community, aware of the problems of the inflammatory state, constantly searches for drugs to remove inflammation. Blood, stool, urine, and saliva tests also exist to find bacteria, viruses, parasites, fungi, and chemical disturbances. Causes overlooked by these tests are food allergies, chemical sensitivities, and free radicals and AGEs, all discussed in depth in Chapters 3 and 4.

The next chapter deals with the healthy state our body should be in—homeostasis, a balanced body chemistry—and reveals how upset body chemistry can cause symptoms, inflammation, and a suppressed immune system.

3 1833 04712 5585

2

Homeostasis– Balanced Body Chemistry

Walter B. Cannon, PhD, MD, (1871–1945) was a Harvard University cum laude graduate, head of the physiology department at Harvard for many years, writer, researcher, and lecturer. He coined the word *homeostasis* in 1932 in his brilliant book, *The Wisdom of the Body.*[1] The basic concept of homeostasis is that it is a biochemical electrical balance in the body that, when present, creates healing. Many bodily systems and properties must remain balanced for homeostasis to occur. Examples of these are the endocrine system (glands that secrete body-regulating hormones), the body's pH (a measurement of acidity/alkalinity), body temperature, and the chemicals in the bloodstream, all of which have precise relationships to each other that should not be altered.

When the body stays out of homeostasis too long and too often, stresses on all other body systems result. Cannon is not alone in his understanding of homeostasis and stress. Some contemporary investigators define stress as "a state of disharmony or threatened homeostasis." During these circumstances, the normal homeostatic mechanisms are superseded by a vast number of changes, resulting in inflammation setting in, and organ systems become compromised.[2] In addition, the digestive system has difficulty digesting and metabolizing food, and the immune system becomes compromised and malfunctions, opening the door to infectious and degenerative diseases.

HOMEOSTASIS REGULATORS

The endocrine system is an important body regulator composed of glands, including the pancreas, the thyroid, the adrenal gland, and the pituitary gland, among others. These glands secrete hormones into the bloodstream to create homeostasis. Some of these hormones secreted include insulin, thyroxin, adrenalin, pituitary hormones, and sex hormones. Our rigorous and unbalanced lifestyles, rife with distress and abusive foods, have exhausted many of our glands, causing extra work and energy expenditures to maintain the delicate balance. Those who suffer such imbalances must rely on insulin for a deficient pancreas, thyroxin for an exhausted thyroid, and adrenalin for depleted adrenal glands.[3] Women with premenstrual and postmenopausal problems due to malfunctioning female sex hormones require a cocktail of estrogen and progesterone, neither of which would be necessary if the body had maintained homeostasis on a regular basis.

Chemicals that flow through the bloodstream, including minerals, vitamins, glucose, cholesterol, blood urea nitrogen, high density lipoproteins, triglycerides, and many others, help to regulate homeostasis.[4] When we eat abusive food, and think, feel, and speak negatively, we deplete our minerals, changing important mineral relationships. Minerals act as the buffers of the body, helping to stabilize the pH, which needs to stay slightly alkaline to function properly. When our blood, saliva, and/or urine become too acidic or alkaline, our body has to work hard to bring it back to the mild alkaline state. We can deplete sodium, potassium, and calcium in order to balance the pH, because the body will do anything to regain and maintain homeostasis. Thermal regulators kick in when a person gets sick with a cold or flu. Body temperature rises in order to kill off the offending virus or bacteria, returning to normal only when the danger is over. As Cannon sagely states, "the body has wisdom." If any of these systems stay out of homeostasis too long, the immune system becomes compromised and the body ages.

PATHWAYS TO UPSET HOMEOSTASIS

The body can unknowingly ingest harmful chemicals, germs, and radioactivity through just about any bodily orifice, such as the mouth, nose, skin, ears, or sex organs. This is all possible. But what we do to ourselves on a daily basis by what we put into our mouths and what comes out of our mouths is the most important aspect of health.

Basically, the two main pathways to change body chemistry and disrupt homeostasis are the mouth and the mind. Abusive foods, such as sugar, overcooked protein, fried foods, hydrogenated fats, food containing too many chemicals, and foods to which our body reacts (individual food allergies), upset our body chemistry. When the psychological stress in our life becomes *distress,* similar effects on our body chemistry occur. Commonly, these chemical changes express themselves as an alteration in the relationships between minerals. No mineral is an island, as they function only in relation to each other. If one mineral becomes depleted in the bloodstream, other minerals can become non-functioning and/or toxic.

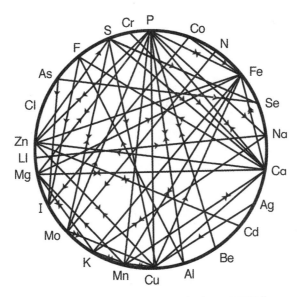

FIGURE 2.1. MINERAL RELATIONSHIP WHEEL[5]
As this wheel shows, each mineral depends on other minerals to function properly.

Dr. Paul Eck, Analytical Research Labs, Phoenix, Arizona

Calcium and phosphorus give structure to our bodies through the formation of bones and teeth. However, most minerals function primarily as enzyme catalysts within cells and body fluids, helping our bodies grow, perform maintenance, regulate our body processes, and supply energy. Very slight changes from normal may result in profound physiological consequences. A person can experience many symptoms or possibly none, without making an appreciable difference in the total mineral makeup of the body.[6]

Digestion needs enzymes to function properly. Enzymes need minerals to function properly. If we have depleted some of the minerals due to upset body chemistry, not all of the foods we eat will digest properly. Food that is not digested and assimilated is acted on in other ways: carbohydrates ferment, proteins putrefy, and fats become rancid. Such changes are caused by bacteria living in the digestive tract that produce by-products called cadaverines, purines, and phenols, all of which have been linked to cancer, among other diseases. These by-products irritate the intestinal mucosa, and can sicken gut bacteria. When 300 to 400 different bacteria species are damaged, a condition called dysbiosis results, which is characterized by an overgrowth of *Candida albicans*, a normally harmless yeast-like fungus inhabiting most humans. This overgrowth causes deterioration of the intestinal wall, allowing other pathogens and partially digested food into the bloodstream.[7]

Nearly 91 million Americans suffer from yeast overgrowth, primarily caused by antibiotics, birth control pills, alcohol, food allergies that inflame the colon, and excess sugar in the diet. *Candida* lives on the moist dark mucous membranes lining the mouth, vagina, and intestinal tract. Ordinarily, the immune system and other competing microorganisms serve to keep yeast colonies small and harmless. But when the delicate balance of the body is tipped, rapid and aggressive growth causes many unpleasant symptoms, some lethal, to the host.

Common expressions of *Candida* overgrowth include vaginal yeast infections, thrush (a white yeast infection of the mouth and tongue common in infants), dandruff, and intense cravings, especially for sweet and starchy foods (yeast's best food source). Such cravings have been linked to overeating and weight gain, chronic fatigue, irritable bowel syndrome, gas, bloating, rashes, mold allergies, slowed mental functioning, depression, painful joints, chronic fungus growths, and symptoms that mimic food allergies.

Dr. William Philpott, in his book *Brain Allergies*, says, "One of the most important systemic functions of the pancreas is to supply proteolytic enzymes (pancreatic enzymes that aid food digestion). These enzymes also act as regulatory mechanisms over inflammatory reactions in the body. Poor digestion of food occurs as a consequence of insufficient pancreatic proteolytic enzymes." As a result, unusable food particles are absorbed through the intestinal mucosa and circulate in the blood, reaching tissues in partially digested form.[8]

Leaky gut syndrome, gut permeability, and intestinal permeability are names the medical community has given for what Philpott described. Partially digested foods are not broken down completely into their simplest forms in the small intestines because of lack of enzymes. Proteins do not digest into amino acids, carbohydrates do not break down into simple sugars, and fats do not become fatty acids. Specific foods, identified by the individual body as harmful (even ones thought of as nutritious and beneficial) can enter the bloodstream when the body chemistry is unbalanced and food digests poorly.

This is a form of food allergy. The body treats such partially digested molecules in the bloodstream as invaders. The immune system tries to protect the body and establishes inflammation around these invaders in a given organ or tissue.[9]

No correlation seems to exist between a specific food and a specific condition. One person can sneeze while eating an apple. Another person can get swollen ankles after eating wheat. Different foods, healthy for some, can cause symptoms and disease in others. All reactive foods must be removed for the afflicted person to heal. Healing time will vary depending on the person involved and the severity of his or her symptoms. An arthritic person's symptoms can disappear in just a few days while someone with psoriasis may take weeks. Skin problems take longer to heal than many other problems.

Absorption of this partially digested food across the human gastrointestinal (GI) mucosal wall and into the bloodstream is commonly known as food allergy. Some of the primary factors that cause or contribute to food allergy include:

- Alcohol abuse.

- Bottle feeding or feeding a baby food during the first six months of life.

- Premature birth.

- Use of non-steroidal anti-inflammatory drugs and other over-the-counter and pharmaceutical drugs.

- Ingestion of all forms of simple sugar, fried food, and hydrogenated fats.

- Gastrointestinal microorganism infection.

- Yeast infections (*Candida albicans*).

- Eating too much food at one sitting (you only have so many enzymes).

As mentioned above, partially digested food and the attendant inflammation can go anywhere in the body and cause problems. In joints or tissues we call this inflammation arthritis, but in the nerves we call it multiple sclerosis. Alternately, such inflammatory particles can go to the face, setting off classic allergy symptoms like sinusitis, runny nose, scratchy throat and ears, ear infections, swollen eyes, and headaches. Not even the brain is immune to inflammation. For years, researchers thought there was a blood-brain barrier (BBB), making it difficult for any foreign particle to get to the brain, but now current research has changed their minds. Foreign particles that reach the brain can cause migraine headaches, anger, fatigue, depression, schizophrenia, and other problems. (See Chapter 5.)

The immune system is capable of removing this foreign invader, this partially digested food, but it was not designed to do this repeatedly. When forced to do so, it becomes exhausted, opening the door to infectious and degenerative diseases. Food allergy is relentless. With or without symptoms, destruction awaits as reactive foods put a continual strain on the immune system, leading to disease and even death. Compounding the problem is the fact that many sufferers of food allergy are unaware that they are affected by it, or that it is affecting their health. The good news is that when you eliminate reactive foods, including junk food, AGEs, and free radicals (see Chapter 4), and do not let stress become distress, the symptoms will go away, and the body will heal.

USING BODY CHEMISTRY

Based on clinical evidence, Philpott observed that a person with an infection is more susceptible to food allergies.[10] He is right. When you have a cold or any germ (an example of upset body chemistry), eat as little as possible because the food will not digest well, causing food allergies and complicating your illness. Forget the old saying, "Feed a cold and starve a fever." The correct advice is to starve a cold *and* starve a fever. Animals do not eat when they are sick, and neither should you. Green juices and lemon water will do for a few days. Give your immune system a chance to deal with the infection.

A recurring sickness should cause you to reevaluate the problem, as it might be the work of an allergen rather than a virus or bacteria. An allergy complete with stuffed up sinuses can change into a full-blown cold as an opportunistic microbe exploits an immune system compromised by allergies.[11] Philpott believes that "there are no tissues or organs in the human body that are free from an assortment of varying types of latent opportunist microorganisms."[12] In homeostasis our microbes live happily and do no damage, but when the body moves out of homeostasis microbial revenge lurks. While many doctors now agree with Philpott, Louis Pasteur's competing theory of a sterile body, where no microbes live, has been the cornerstone of medical thought for the past century. Consequent neglect of research into homeostasis and what causes microbes to turn against us may have caused much harm for many people.

CONCLUSION

While our genetic blueprint may illustrate what sickness we may get, our lifestyle determines *if* we'll get sick at all. In my extensive travels to developing nations, I have talked to health practitioners who report that the incidence of modern diseases is low. The absence of most degenerative disease in developing nations should be a milestone for instruction in the disease process. In the western world, sick people are studied to find out cures for disease instead of studying healthy people to find out why they are healthy. I hope that the study of homeostasis and balanced body chemistry will be in the medical school curriculum soon.

In the next chapter, we will examine how allergies and sensitivities can contribute to inflammation.

3

Allergies and Inflammation

Research has shown that there is a strong link between inflammation and allergies and sensitivities. Moreover, inflammation is typically part of the body's response to allergic reactions. Allergies and sensitivities fall into two categories—food allergies and environmental allergies, including multiple chemical sensitivities. In this chapter, we will examine how both types of allergies can cause inflammation, and what you can do to prevent and reverse allergies. (For additional information about how you can test for allergies, see Chapter 6.)

FOOD ALLERGY

Allergic diseases have reached epidemic proportions in the United States. This widespread condition affects nearly 30 percent of the population of most developed countries, according to Dr. Marc Rothenberg, section chief of allergy and clinical immunology at Cincinnati Children's Hospital.[1] Dr. R. Forman, author of *How to Control Your Allergies*, asserts that 30–100 million people suffer from allergies, making them the costliest health care problem today.[2] Another estimate says that as many as 60 percent of the population suffers from undetected food allergies.[3]

Symptoms like sneezing, wheezing, itching, diarrhea, or other gastrointestinal conditions are commonly associated with allergy. However, you might not have any of these classic symptoms of food allergy but still be adversely affected by food. Presented on the following page is a more complete list of food allergy symptoms.

Physical Symptoms of Food Allergies

Abdominal pain
Aching muscles
Acne
Addictions
Anemia
Arthritis
Asthma
Athlete's foot
Bad breath
Bed-wetting
Blackouts
Bloating
Blood sugar
  problems
Bloody stools
Blurred vision
Breast pain
Bursitis
Canker sores
Celiac disease
Chronic bladder
  infections
Chronic fatigue
  syndrome
Chronic or recurrent
  infections
Coated tongue
Colitis
Compulsive drinking
Constant hunger
Constipation
Coughing
Cravings for certain
  foods
Difficulty in
  swallowing
Dizziness
Eczema
Excessive thirst
Excessive or no
  sweating
Failure of newborn
  infants to develop

Fainting
Fatigue
Feeling drained
Flushes
Frequent need to
  urinate
Gall bladder disease
Gas
Gastritis
Gritty feeling in eyes
Headaches, all types
Heavy body odor
High/low blood
  pressure
Hives
Hyperactivity
Indigestion—
  recurring
Infant colic
Inflammation
Insomnia
Intestinal bleeding
Irritability
Irritable Bowel
  Syndrome
Itching
Itchy or red eyes
  and/or ears
Lethargy
Loss of appetite
Lower back pain
Malabsorption of
  food
Menstrual
  problems
Metallic taste
Mouth ulcers
Multiple sclerosis
  (MS)
Muscle aches and
  cramps
Muscle tremors

Nausea
Palpitations
Persistent cough
Poor balance
Postnasal drip
Premenstrual
  problems
Racing pulse
Rashes
Recurrent bronchitis
Recurrent croup
Recurrent ear
  infections
Restless legs
  syndrome
Rhinitis
Schizophrenia
Seizures
Sensitivity to light
  and noise
Sinusitis
Sleep disturbances
Sore tongue
Sore, itching, puffy
  or burning eyes
Stiff neck
Styes
Systemic Lupus
  Erythematosus
  (SLE)
Temperature
  fluctuations
Thrush
Tics
Tenets
Ulcerative colitis
Ulcers
Vertigo
Vomiting
Watering eyes
Weight gain or loss
Wheezing[4]

The inflammatory process can cause any of these symptoms. A person who has these ailments usually takes an anti-inflammatory or antihistamine pill, controlling the symptoms but not the causes. The person with symptoms is the lucky one, because he or she understands something is wrong, but the person without symptoms has no idea that a food can cause a degenerative disease later in life. Such a person is probably unaware that allergies weaken the immune system, creating a greater susceptibility to colds and other infectious diseases, as well as degenerative diseases.

Food allergy, defined as a complex of syndromes resulting from a body sensitizing to one or more foods, occurs when the immune system recognizes an otherwise harmless food as hostile. This mobilization of the body's defenses causes symptoms of allergy and the resulting inflammation. Reactions range from not feeling anything, to mildly inconvenient and uncomfortable symptoms, to total failure of the organ(s) that are unable to be protected by the immune system.

Somewhere between discomfort and organ failure lie more violent reactions. Under continued stress and lack of homeostasis, when the immune system misidentifies and reacts to a food, the response occurs with a ferocity that is far greater than required. It is only then that many people become aware of their allergies. "The problem is not that 25% of people recognize symptoms from food ingestion, but that many more people do not recognize that food is making them ill."[5]

Celiac disease (gluten intolerance) is a demonstrative example of how food reactions can produce serious diseases. It is one of many unsolved ailments of our civilization that is inflammatory and related to immune response. The reason it is unsolved is because many more people than are diagnosed have a gluten intolerance to some degree but are not aware of it. (More information on inflammatory bowel diseases and celiac disease is presented in Chapter 5.)

Consider a description of a food allergy in the writings of the ancient Greek physician, Hippocrates, more than 2,000 years ago:

> But there are persons who cannot readily change their diet with impunity; and if they make any alteration in it for one day, or even a part of a day, are greatly injured thereby. Such persons, provided they take dinner when it is not their wont, immediately become heavy and inactive, both in mind and body, and are weighed down with yawning, slumbering, and thirst; and if they take supper in addition, they are seized with flatulence,

termini, and diarrhea, and to many this has been the commencement of serious disease, when they have merely taken twice in a day the same food which they have been in the custom of taking once.

It seems from Hippocrates' clinical description that patient complaints have not changed in the millennia since he lived. Observation shows that similar foods cause widely varied symptoms among large samples of people. Such reactions are determined by an individual's genetic blueprint that even governs how often a food can be eaten without causing problems. Some can eat a food once a day, but can not eat that food more often, others can only eat that same food once in four days and still others cannot eat the food at all. It follows that repeated exposure to food allergens compound problems and provoke severe symptoms.

One form of this repeated exposure comes from overeating and eating when you are not hungry. So follow Hippocrates' advice. Eat only when you are hungry, and eat small portions, taking care to eliminate the foods to which you react.

Food Allergy and Food Hypersensitivity

Every book and medical journal that is written on food allergy has a variation on what the definition is, but the one presented below will suffice. I will detail how the medical community has defined food allergy and food sensitivity, while presenting my opinions of these definitions.

Food Allergy

In the past, "allergy" was a name given when a person reacted with a specific antibody called IgE (immunoglobulin E), to a substance during a RAST blood test, or to a skin prick test (see Chapter 6). When food was tested and a person reacted, doctors named the condition immediate-onset, IgE-mediated and/or atopic food allergy. Allergists noticed three members of the atopic group: hay fever (seasonal allergic rhinitis and conjunctivitis), asthma, and eczema. Doctors quickly adopted the IgE model as the sole explanation of allergy because testing for sensitization was simple. Under this model, only a few people, estimated at less than five percent of the population, primarily children, have allergies.

When partially-digested food leaks into the bloodstream where it does not belong, the immune system sends antibodies to deal with the situation. The immune system does this because partially-digested food in the bloodstream can be toxic. Of the many types of antibodies the body produces, only IgE reacts to this type of food allergy problem, setting up a situation where the body will continuously react the same way when the food is again eaten.

One side of the antibody recognizes the food and binds to it, while the other side will attach to a mast cell, another type of immune cell. Mast cells release inflammation-causing histamine, kinins, cytokines, prostaglandins, and other allergy-related chemicals at any point in their journey through the body. The offending food, an antibody, and a mast cell make up a circulating immune complex (CIC). The CIC may not react in the gastrointestinal tract but may react in the blood or target organs, especially the lungs and connective tissue. Usually this type of allergy strikes immediately or shortly after consumption of the suspect food. This causes obvious allergic reactions, such as sneezing, rapid breathing, skin rashes, burning throat, acute abdominal pain, vomiting, and/or diarrhea.[6] An IgE response is immediate and the symptoms are loud and clear, making it easy to diagnose.

The IgE model has not always been successful explaining inflammatory reactions to food, however. Some people with many symptoms test negative to foods using the IgE test, continue to eat the food, and continue to have symptoms. Others only receive partial results because all the food allergies have not been detected.

Claiming that the IgE blood test or skin prick test are the only valid tests for allergies seems to ignore a plethora of other possible explanations. A better way to look at the problems a person has with a food is to look at *both* the immediate reaction and the delayed reaction that can signal chronic immune weakness. The delayed reaction does not fall into the IgE model and is more difficult to test.

Food Hypersensitivity

Immune reactions to food take other forms than IgE responses. Rather than being called an allergy, such reactions are often termed food hypersensitivity, food intolerance, food idiosyncrasy, food metabolic reaction, masked food allergy, food toxicity reaction or syndrome, maladaptive response or reaction, or hidden food allergy.[7] An IgE blood test will not recognize any of these reactions.

Food hypersensitivity is an immune response that is much more common than food allergy. It involves a different immunoglobulin mediator than IgE, usually IgG (immunoglobulin G), but sometimes the other immunoglobulins: IgA, IgD, or IgM. Unlike IgE, IgG does not bind to mast cells. Instead, it attaches itself directly to the food as it enters the bloodstream, forming a different type of CIC. Delays of two hours to several days for reactions after consuming IgG-reactive foods have been recorded.

Delayed food reactions can be responsible for a wide variety of complaints that, at first glance, lack a plausible explanation, yet still cause varied symptoms, as shown in the chart on the next page. Paradoxically, the person with an IgG response can be addicted to the food, feeling better in the wake of consumption, only to feel chronic symptoms hours or days later. In this case, medical histories and diet diaries become useless for ferreting out hidden allergies. When a symptom occurs a few hours or a few days after eating a food, it is difficult to figure out what food caused the symptom.

Since reactions are similar and adverse conditions can occur whether the reactions are IgG-mediated, IgE-mediated, or due to any other reaction, the term *allergy* will be used throughout this book for any adverse reaction that takes place anywhere in the body due to a food.

How long do allergies of both types last? Does a person have these allergies for a lifetime? Most IgE-mediated reactions are permanent, as are some IgG-mediated conditions, which are usually the result of extensive immune system abuse. My personal experience with my allergies suggests that two months of complete abstinence from the allergic food is the minimum required to clear a normal IgG allergy. Abnormally intense allergies (for me, triggered by onions) will take longer (for me, six months), depending upon the correlation of genetics and immune system damage. If an allergy clears, the person may resume eating the food provided homeostasis is maintained, which can be tested for with my Body Monitor Kit. (See page 128.)

I must stress complete abstinence from allergy-inducing food and sugar while the body heals. *Everybody* reacts adversely to sugar. Sugar so upsets the body chemistry that it can cause new allergies, so not removing sugar from your diet will waste your

A COMPARISON OF THE DIFFERENCES BETWEEN ALLERGY (Immediate Reaction) AND HYPERSENSITIVITY (Delayed Reaction)

IMMEDIATE REACTION	DELAYED REACTION
Rarely more than a few foods are involved.	Multiple foods can be involved.
Small amount of food can cause severe reaction.	Small or sometimes large amounts of the food can cause a reaction.
Reactions occur 2 hours or less after consumption of offending foods.	Reactions occur 2-24 hours after eating offending foods; rarely up to 72 hours have reactions been reported.
Primarily effects: Skin, airway, and digestive system.	Any organ system can be involved in reaction.
Rare in adults.	Very common in children and adults.
Addictive cravings never seen.	Addictive cravings and withdrawal seen in 20-30 percent of cases.
Offending food is often diagnosed because of immediate reaction.	Because of multiple foods and delayed onset of symptoms, the offending foods are rarely self-diagnosed.
Allergic food is a rarely eaten food.	Allergic foods are favorite foods a person craves.
A permanent fixed allergy.	Many symptoms clear after avoidance for a few months (a different time for each person).
IgE and skin test: positive reaction.	IgE negative; IgG positive often.
Mast cell release of histamine and tryptase involved.	Sensitized lymphocytes, eosinophils, platelets, release of leukotrienes prevalent.
When people quit eating foods that cause symptoms, they have no withdrawal or delayed food allergy detoxification symptoms; they do not crave or miss these foods.	Powerful addictive cravings and disabling immediate symptoms are reported in over 30 percent of patients when they stop eating the reactive food.

time. Everyone responds differently when suspect foods are eliminated from their diet. Allergies will clear shortly for some, and for
others more time is needed. See page 127 for information on how
to test for food allergies.

Most Common Foods to Which a Person Reacts

Barley	Eggs	Sugar
Beef	Nuts	(all forms)*
Chocolate	Peanuts	Tea
Citrus	Rye	Tomatoes
Coffee	Seafood	Wheat
Dairy	Soy	Yeast

*Everyone reacts to sugar, although an allergy test might not disclose this.

A person can also react to other foods not included in the above
list, because anything that goes in the mouth, including vitamins,
minerals, herbs, homeopathic drugs, or other supplements, can be
a problem. What you crave is likely to be to what you react. Philpott
believes that the foods to which a person reacts are specific for that
individual and so are the symptoms that occur.[8] Further information on food additives that may also contribute to the problem is
presented later in this chapter. A useful rule of thumb among food
allergy experts is that for every food identified to be allergy-
induced, two more go undiagnosed, and at least one more assessment will be wrong.[9]

Food Allergy and Inflammation

In the past, prevailing theory held that mast cells were the major
cause of inflammation. An ingested allergen can cause eosinophils to
invade gastrointestinal tissues, creating difficulty in moving food
through the GI tract, inflammation, and enlargement of the stomach,
according to Dr. Rothenberg. "Allergies do affect the GI tract; they're
serious, and eosinophils are the culprits. Oral antigens—foods that
people are allergic to—induce eosinophilic inflammation in various
segments of the gastrointestinal tract, including the esophagus, stomach, and small intestine."[10]

Eosinophils are immune cells packed with powerful proteins that destroy surrounding tissues and rally other immune cells to infections. Eosinophils can appear in high numbers at sites of allergic reaction. They cause the walls of digestive organs to swell and food becomes stalled in the stomach. The eosinophils attack healthy tissue and cause disease, perhaps damaging the nerve cells that communicate with the digestive tract.[11]

When we are healthy, our immune system ignores our food, but when we are unhealthy, the immune system rushes in and creates allergies. In one of Rothenberg's studies, he made animals allergic to certain foods. The animals became ill and lost weight as multiple regions of their digestive tracts experienced inflammation caused by immune cells rushing to the affected areas. Eosinophils accumulated in high numbers, particularly around damaged nerve cells, and the walls of digestive organs swelled, and food became stalled in the stomach. Both of these findings are characteristic of human eosinophilic gastrointestinal inflammation.[12]

Leaky Gut Syndrome, Gut Permeability

Not only can the GI tract become inflamed, so can the bloodstream. In the case of leaky gut syndrome, the epithelium (the lining of the intestine) on the villi (wavy-like fingers) of the small intestine becomes inflamed and irritated, allowing metabolic and microbial toxins to flood the bloodstream. Once the gut develops these large leaky spaces, toxins escape to overload the liver, causing unpleasant conditions and degenerative diseases associated with aging.[13] These toxins, chemicals, foods, AGEs (see page 39), free radicals, pharmaceutical drugs, over-the-counter drugs, or infectious agents move through the leaky gut mucosa, creating systemic inflammation anywhere in the body. Among other problems, this irritation causes a failure of intestinal defense mechanisms leading to multiple organ failure and death in critically ill patients.[14]

We constantly irritate the lining of our digestive tract with high intake of sugars, food additives, herbicide-pesticide residues, alcohol,[15] caffeine, dangerous bacterial strains, FDA-approved drugs, over-the-counter drugs, and street drugs. Leaky gut syndrome results from the constant damage from all of these inflammatory processes, whether it is antibiotics killing friendly bacteria that control *Candida*, or food allergies wiping out the digestive tract.

Psychological Stress

It has long been known that stress affects both the stomach and colon, as shown by the very high prevalence of gastrointestinal symptoms among patients with psychiatric illness. Eating when stressed can result in poorly digested food, which can escape into the bloodstream, causing food allergy and affecting any cell, tissue, gland, or organ in the body.[16] (See Chapter 4 for more information on stress.)

Food allergy plays a far greater role in the degenerative disease process than has been recognized previously, although medical literature has acknowledged it for many years. Finding the foods to which your body reacts is a matter of taking two blood tests. One tests for IgE immediate reactions, and the other tests for IgG delayed reactions. You will need to talk to your health care provider to find a blood lab that does these tests. Not all blood labs do these tests. It is important to do both. Removing food allergens can be a lifesaver.

ENVIRONMENTAL ILLNESS

(Chemical Sensitivities; Multiple Chemical Sensitivities (MCS); Multiple, Environmental and Seasonal Allergies; Environmental Sensitivity; Environmentally Triggered Illnesses (EI); Ecological Illness; Idiopathic Environmental Intolerance; Total Allergic Syndrome; Total Immune Disorder Syndrome)

Environmental illness, or chemical sensitivities, can be defined as any adverse reaction to chemicals in our air, food, and water, generally accepted as nontoxic. It is a chronic condition that is characterized by multiple symptoms, in multiple organs, affecting multiple senses, and triggered by multiple chemicals. The most common reactions are headache, fatigue, dizziness, nausea, memory problems, breathing problems, flu-like symptoms, rashes, and hives. Usually the symptoms fade between exposures, but some people have the symptoms all the time.

Environmental illness results when the body becomes unable to adapt to toxins and maintain homeostasis. Disruption may result from a wide range of possible exposures. The insult can be caused by a severe acute exposure, cumulative low-grade exposures, and/or multiple stressors over time. Symptoms are determined by type of stressor, timing of exposure, individual biochemistry, and the condition of the person.[17]

People affected by environmental illness describe not being able to stand in line behind someone wearing perfume without getting a severe headache, or to walk through the laundry detergent aisle in the supermarket without having trouble breathing, or being unable to pump gas because they feel dizzy and nauseous. Numerous other symptoms and difficulties may also be involved.

Among the general population, exposure to chemicals might not be diagnosed as chemical sensitivity, but this exposure can cause adverse effects, nonetheless. A long-term study with more than 500,000 people demonstrated the disease risks of breathing polluted air. The researchers linked particles deep in the lungs and the presence of sulphur oxides to an increased risk of dying from lung cancer or various cardiopulmonary diseases, including heart attack, stroke, asthma, pneumonia, and chronic obstructive pulmonary diseases like emphysema and bronchitis. More importantly, *the death rate from any cause also rose when pollution levels increased.*[18] Passing ordinances and regulations to clean the air and water are the first steps towards becoming healthy. In the meantime, included below are some personally achievable solutions for dealing with environmental toxins.

What Causes Environmental and Seasonal Allergies?

Most people with chemical, seasonal, and/or exercise-induced allergies also have food allergies (see above). For many, food allergies can be too low-grade to be felt directly, or may be masked by the environmental symptoms.[19] At certain times of the year, pollens and other environmental factors can cause rhinitis (nasal congestion and obstruction, sneezing, nasal and palate itching, diminished smell and hearing, generalized itching, and headaches). Other symptoms of seasonal allergies include allergic conjunctivitis (red eyes) and vernal keratoconjunctivitis (red, swollen and watery eyes). Such symptoms represent an overloaded immune system that is breaking down under great insult, creating inflammation as it attempts to heal.

Most allergists believe that all allergy symptoms, especially rhinitis, are solely caused by inhalant or environmental allergies. Many times this is not the case, however. In a study of 197 patients with year-round rhinitis, tests for food allergy and food additives came back positive in most cases for many substances. Eliminating the substances drove away the complaints thought to be inhalant-based.[20]

I am an excellent example of this phenomenon. Living in Los Angeles, I used to run and hide in my room from the hot Santa Ana winds that brought pollen and dust with them. My non-airtight room would not protect me, and I would suffer through twenty-four hours of sneezing, watery eyes, and various degrees of inflammation. Realizing that I was concurrently allergic to various foods, I eliminated them and the junk foods to which everyone reacts. In time, as my body healed and I reintegrated most of the allergy foods into my diet, my problems with a windy day diminished to the point of nothingness. My immune system is now strong enough to deal with the pollen and dust. Remove the foods to which you react and the inhalant allergies will go away.[21]

Dr. Joseph Mercola, founder of the popular Internet health site, www.mercola.com, made this same discovery. He found that inhaled allergies dissipated after changing an eight-year-old girl's diet to whole foods without any sugar, dairy, or wheat. The girl previously took multiple shots for inhalant allergies that caused her asthma. Although Mercola wanted to give a food allergy test, he was unable to because the child had been so traumatized by needle sticks. Her symptoms and reliance on inhalers or shots diminished greatly within eighteen months.

Removing just the wheat, dairy, and sugar took enough of a load off of her system to heal the immune system within a year and a half. Mercola found that when the girl goes off of her diet her symptoms return.[22] I feel if he had been able to test her for food allergies and removed those other foods to which she reacted, the healing would have taken far less time.

Allergy to Inhaled Food Allergens

Smelling a food allergen while it cooks can also trigger allergic responses. In a fascinating study, researchers identified children with a food allergy who developed asthma in the presence of an odor. The researchers exposed subjects in a small kitchen for twenty minutes to the aerosolized form of different allergens, while monitoring symptoms. The children developed asthma and decreased respiratory function in the presence of fish, chickpeas, milk, eggs, and/or buckwheat, but did not react to seven different other food items.[23]

The methodology of this experiment is somewhat limited since more food odors could have been tested. Other research suggests that some asthmatic children will not react at all to odors. However, the results *do* indicate a general linkage that must be taken into account when treating environmental allergies.

Germs and Environmental Allergies

There is also a relationship between infections and new food allergies. Dr. William Spannhake, associate chairman of the Department of Environmental Health Sciences at Johns Hopkins University, found that infectious viruses and pollutants prompt kinins that release inflammatory agents, making people feel sick. Food allergy stimulates the same responses, so when a virus and airborne chemicals are added, the total wreckage is greater than the sum of parts. "We found that these two stimuli, which on the surface appear to be quite different, lead to the same type of increase in inflammation. This can be very detrimental to a person who has asthma and a low-grade inflammation at all times," says Spannhake.[24]

Previously, I suggested that total abstinence from allergic foods for a time was required for healing. This is also true for chemicals and inhalants. The immune system needs a chance to heal after being overloaded with reactive foods, chemicals, inhalants, and a variety of infectious vectors. Failure to make these changes may allow symptoms to continue.

Many times when you go to a dentist or a doctor, he or she asks if you are allergic to any pharmaceutical drugs. Many know they have an allergy to a drug but others are unaware. This is because not all reactions are immediate, with some not manifesting until seven to ten days after exposure. A general course of detoxification and a few weeks of taking probiotics that replace helpful bacteria after taking pharmaceutical drugs are good ideas. (See Chapters 7 and 8.)

Food Additives

Over the years, people have reported to the Food and Drug Administration (FDA) many adverse reactions to food additives, including migraines, edema (swelling), rashes, asthma, and angioedema (swollen arteries). Aspartame (a sweetener), monosodium glutamate (a flavor enhancer), sulfur-based preservatives, and tartrazine, also known as FD&C Yellow No. 5 (a food color) are the biggest culprits, along with benzoic acid parabens.

Sulfites

Every day, the use of sulfur in the American food industry grows. Sulfites and sulfur dioxide preservatives are most noticeable in wine, dried fruit, instant potatoes, French fries, pizza, cold drinks, and fruit juice concentrates. Sprayed onto foods to keep them fresh and prevent discoloration, sulfites also find their way into cold cuts and salads. They are also hidden in hundreds of ingredients like corn syrup and gelatin, which are contained in thousands of other food products.

The FDA uses the term "allergic-type responses" to describe the range of symptoms suffered by these individuals after eating sulfite-treated foods. These chemicals, in the form of gases, cause lung irritation and may trigger asthma, with responses ranging from mild to life-threatening. To help sulfite-sensitive people avoid problems, the FDA requires the presence of sulfites in processed foods to be declared on the label, and prohibits their use on fresh produce intended to be sold or served raw to consumers. Chemicals in this class include sulphur dioxide, sodium sulfite, sodium bisulfite, potassium bisulfite, and potassium metasulfite.

Benzoic acid and Parabens

Benzoates and parabens have antibacterial and antifungal properties to prevent food spoilage. These agents are added to pharmaceutical and food products, and occur naturally in prunes, cinnamon, tea, and berries. Hives, asthma, and angioedema are the most common symptoms of ingestion of these substances. Words to look out for on food and package labels include benzoic acid, sodium benzoate, methylparaben, propylparaben, and heptylparaben. To avoid these substances altogether, eat only whole foods that are unpackaged.

Antioxidants

Fat and oils in food turn rancid when exposed to air. Synthetic phenolic antioxidants, butylated hydroxyanisole (BHA), and butylated hydroxytoluene (BHT) prevent this from happening but can trigger asthma, rhinitis, and urticaria, as well as many other symptoms.

Remember to keep your fats and oils in the refrigerator and your nuts and seeds in the freezer.

Aspartame and other Flavor Additives and Sweeteners

Aspartame, a low-calorie sweetener that can trigger many different symptoms in people, contains two normal amino acids: phenylalanine and aspartic acid. After reviewing scientific studies in 1981, the FDA determined that aspartame was safe for use in foods. I feel that there is enough evidence to show that aspartame should be avoided altogether.

Certain people with the genetic disease phenylketonuria (PKU) cannot effectively metabolize phenylalanine. Nor can people with advanced liver disease, or pregnant women with hyperphenylalanine (high levels of phenylalanine in their blood). High levels of this amino acid in body fluids can cause brain damage, heralded by seizures, dizziness, tremors, migraines, memory loss, slurred speech, and confusion.

Other sweeteners that should be avoided are Sucralose (Splenda) and Acesulfame K (Sweet One). For much more information on the toxicity of various sweeteners go to the Aspartame (NutraSweet) Toxicity Center at www.holisticmed.com/aspartame. This site lists all toxic sweeteners, not just aspartame.

Monosodium Glutamate

Monosodium Glutamate (MSG) can trigger the "Chinese Restaurant Syndrome" of burning and tightness in the chest, neck, and face. For some people, that is just the beginning. MSG is "generally recognized as safe, a GRAS product" by the FDA, which has studied the available evidence concerning MSG safety. The agency also has an ongoing contract with the Federation of American Societies for Experimental Biology to re-examine the scientific data on possible adverse reactions to glutamate. MSG must be declared on the label of any food to which it is added. Ask at Chinese restaurants if they use MSG if you have health problems, and even if you do not have health problems. The less chemicals your body has to deal with, the less work it has to do, and the healthier you will be.

Food Coloring

All food colors must now be labeled. Many of them can trigger hives, urticaria, asthma, and generalized allergic reactions in susceptible people. I feel that they should be avoided altogether.

Nitrites

Nitrites, widely used processed-meat preservatives, combine with amino acids in the GI tract, creating potentially cancer-causing molecules known as nitrosamines. Additional sources of nitrites include: bacteria breaking down protein and nitrates (a similar class of preservatives) in the mouth and intestines, some natural occurrence in foods, and various sodium salts. Thankfully the incidence of nitrites in the food supply is relatively low, pegged at 2–3 milligrams per day per person. Even so, the cancer risks of nitrosamines may eventually cause health officials to take a second look at the advisability of using nitrites in foods.

Vitamin C inhibits nitrosamine formation and may protect against GI tract cancers. Since vitamin C is also an antioxidant preservative, replacing nitrate and nitrite preservatives with vitamin C in every food where it will work could go a long way towards preventing cancer. Of course, no amount of vitamin C will help against the massive direct injections of nitrosamines into the body from tobacco smoke, *so don't smoke!*

Of all the various additives in the world, only the most common classes are listed here, but it should make sense that any additive is likely to irritate and inflame some people. Another area of concern with these chemicals is their effect on the liver, which may become toxic and fail to filter substances out of the body. A good rule of thumb is, if you cannot pronounce it or spell it, do not put it in your mouth. I have presented food plans in Chapter 7 that should help in removing chemicals. I recommend Plans II and III for this purpose.

Amines

Amines are naturally occurring, nonadditive compound chemicals in certain foods that can accumulate in the body over time, causing reactions that mimic allergies. For some people, amine sensitivity can be limited to a specific amine such as histamine, phenylethylamine, serotonin, and tyramine. Cooking certain foods, particularly meats, at high temperatures produces a further set of amines that can also cause problems.

If toast does not agree with you it is easy to think that wheat is the problem; if a grilled steak upsets you then you might think you have a problem with beef. But in both cases the problem could be amines. There is no specific list of symptoms indicated for amines but migraines that do not respond to other treatments may be relieved by a diet low in all amines or by specifically avoiding individual amines.

Foods that have a high level of amines include:

Vegetables: Sauerkraut, spinach.

Meat, fish, and poultry: Any form of dried, pickled, salted, or smoked. Anchovies, beef liver, fish roe, meat pies and pasties, processed fish products (such as fish fingers, cakes, paste), salami, sausages, tuna (tinned).

Dairy: Virtually all cheeses.

Sweets: Dark chocolate

Condiments: Hydrolyzed protein, miso, tempeh, yeast extracts.

Beverages: Chocolate-flavored drinks, cocoa, cola drinks, orange juice, tomato juice, vegetable juices.[25]

Salicylates

Salicylates, found in curry, dried herbs, tea, almonds, vegetable and fruit skins, can induce urticaria, asthma, and nasal polyps. Medicinal salicylates form from plant sources such as willow-bark methylsalicylate. As oil of wintergreen, methylsalicylate has been rubbed on many cold-stricken chests and inhaled by coughing children for years.

Acetylsalicylic acid (aspirin) can cause GI tract irritation, bleeding, rashes, and hives. Salicylates also occasionally trigger asthma. Dr. Benjamin Feingold postulated that salicylates and food dyes produced hyperactivity in children, popularizing low-salicylate diets. Feingold recommended avoiding foods that contained natural salicylates or chemically similar substances. He also recommended eliminating artificial colors and flavors; the antioxidants BHA and BHT; and aspirin-containing products. With a small child who has hyperactivity, it would be wise to find out more about this diet and try it for a week. You have nothing to lose, except the child's over-active behavior.[26] I feel that Feingold should have gone one step farther in his diet, by removing sugar from the diet, as well.

Airborne Allergies

You know you blow your nose more at certain times of the year and your nose runs more when you exercise in the early morning: therefore, you think you have airborne allergies. It sounds logical. But before you do any testing for airborne allergies, remove the foods to

Exercise-Induced Allergy

Exercise-induced allergy is a puzzle to most health professionals, as symptoms do not manifest until people engage in exercise. Then noses run and eyes itch, or chest pains result. Symptoms are usually precipitated by moderate-to-hard exercise early in the activity, frequently while jogging in a warm humid environment, though sometimes eating before exercise has been a factor.[27]

My long-ago experiences as a national junior tennis champion may be instructive in explaining the causes of exercise-induced allergies. As someone who figuratively died in the presence of flower pollen, especially hibiscus, going onto the court in a breeze could cause a reaction, but only after some minutes of play, when sneezing and inflammation set in. The body heat of the exercise proved to be a contributing factor. Days with still air proved to be equally harsh, but with or without breezes, the cause was eating an allergic food. Since those dark days, my allergies of all kinds have been greatly reduced as I stopped eating the foods to which I reacted for a few months. Most of the foods that caused a reaction then no longer do so today. Most allergies will go away if you put your body back in homeostasis and let it heal.

Another example of this phenomenon is that some people suffer from heart disease related to chest pains while exercising. A study of sixty patients with such chest pain triggered by exercise—a condition known as stable angina—showed higher levels of macrophages (white blood cells), C-reactive protein (CRP) (a marker of inflammation in the bloodstream), and cytokines (inflammatory proteins secreted by the leukocytes), compared with twenty-four people without angina. Although crucial to fighting infection, the release of cytokines is thought to contribute to heart disease by encouraging deposits of cholesterol in fatty plaques lining the arteries, as well as making the deposits in the coronary arteries prone to rupture—thus causing a heart attack.[28]

which you react and most will find that many of the airborne allergies go away. When you take a load off your immune system by removing foods to which you react, your immune system can deal with pollen, horse dander, and other airborne allergies. So wait two months after removing the offending foods and most people will be able to take a deep breath anywhere.

Chemical Sensitivities

We all breathe in the same air and live among many of the same chemicals, but reactions to these chemicals vary from none at all to anaphylactic shock in different people. A sensitive person exposed to air pollution and other chemicals may experience behavioral changes and reduced psychological well-being. Numerous toxic pollutants can interfere with the development and functioning of the adult nervous system, causing emotional upheaval. If you are exposed to chemicals on a daily basis, you might think of being tested for excessive amounts in your body. People who work in beauty shops (hair and nails), dry cleaning shops, or photographic shops; chemists; painters; miners; and people who remove mold, asbestos, and other toxic materials might have this test. (For how to test for chemical sensitivities, see Chapter 6.)

Agents whose exposures are associated with symptoms, and suspected of causing onset, of chemical sensitivity with chronic illness include gasoline, kerosene, natural gas, pesticides (especially chlordane and chlorpyrifos), solvents, new carpet and other renovation materials, adhesives/glues, fiberglass, carbonless copy paper, fabric softener, formaldehyde and glutaraldehyde, carpet shampoos (lauryl sulfate) and other cleaning agents, isocyanates, combustion products (poorly vented gas heaters, overheated batteries), and medications (dinitrochlorobenzene for warts, intranasally packed neosynephrine, prolonged antibiotics, and general anesthesia with petrochemicals). Many parts of the body can become toxic due to toxic metals. Symptoms can include inflammation (respiratory, gastrointestinal, genitourinary) and other immune activation.[29]

Most of the symptoms in this chapter spring from food allergies, but usually manifest as an environmental symptom. Particles that lodge in lungs, chemicals, pollens, and dust wreak havoc in specific ways, but only after the immune system is made too weak to fight. People with environmental allergies should get a blood test for both

IgE and IgG food allergies and chemical sensitivities and do their best to remove all allergens from their life until healing sets in. Detoxification programs also exist to help people along the path of healing. (See Chapter 8.)

CONCLUSION

As you can see from the information I have presented in this chapter, your health can easily be compromised by inflammation and allergic reactions. These immune responses can be due to the wide variety of chemical agents in both our food supply and environment that can trigger them. Becoming aware of such risk factors and making a commitment to avoid them is a vital first step you need to take in order to protect yourself. Fortunately, there is much you can do in this area to ensure good health, especially following the guidelines and suggestions I provide in Parts Two and Three of this book. First, though, let us move on to Chapter 4, where we will explore other associated causes of inflammation, including the interlinked relationship between psychological stress and brain allergies.

4

Other Causes of Inflammation

There are other primary causes of inflammation that we should explore. These include AGEs (advanced glycation end products), free radical damage and oxidative stress, and psychological stress, all of which are prevalent in our modern world. But, as with food and environmental allergies, once you become aware of them and know what to do to minimize their effects, you become empowered to take back control over your health. Let us examine each of them in turn.

AGEs (Advanced Glycation End Products), GLYCATION, AND GLYCOSYLATION

In 1912, a Frenchman, Louis Maillard, investigated the browning and toughening that occurred when foods were cooked. He discovered that glucose (sugar) attached to protein in an abnormal way. Called the Maillard Reaction, this process causes toast to brown and steak to toughen at high temperatures. Maillard also found that the protein changed structure, creating a situation where an unrecognizable new food class could not be digested, assimilated, or metabolized in the body. Barbequing and frying can also cause the Maillard Reaction. Food scientists continue to research the Maillard Reaction, trying to isolate these newly formed proteins, which are also found in processed food, because recent evidence links it to cancer. Though research is ongoing, in the meantime, it makes sense to avoid eating foods that cause the reaction, given the negative health effects they can provoke.

Sugar is one of these foods. Research shows that elevated blood glucose, common after ingesting sugar, can cause the same reaction with proteins in the body.[1] We eat over 158 pounds of sugar per person per year in the United States.[2] Such a sugar glut can cause more people's blood glucose to shoot through the roof than in the past, when less sugar was generally consumed. Under these conditions, where the bloodstream is swimming in sugar, sugars and proteins bind non-enzymatically. But sugar and protein are not supposed to bind non-enzymatically. When they do, the product that is formed is called glycated protein or advanced glycation end products (AGEs). Additionally, sugar can form AGEs with fats, RNA, and DNA.[3]

Normally, sugar binds enzymatically to protein in our body to form glycoproteins, which are essential to proper body functioning. All such reactions are under strict enzyme control and tight metabolic regulation, following predetermined patterns of activity to achieve specific goals.

Copper is depleted when food is overcooked and when protein and sugar combine to form AGEs. As stated before, when there is not enough of a mineral, body chemistry becomes upset, throwing the body out of homeostasis. Therefore, the mineral-dependent enzymes cannot function and the sugar and protein cannot bind in their natural way with enzymes. Deficiency of copper in the diet further allows non-enzymatic bonding between sugars and proteins, causing AGEs.[4]

Altering this process to a non-enyzmatic binding can permanently change the molecular structure of protein and upset proper body function. Protein turns toxic, becoming an invader rather than a helper, and inflammation creeps in, causing decreased cellular function, and an exhausted immune system. The resulting degeneration takes place over time, starting as minor disturbances or disabilities and later developing into serious illnesses.

Protein glycation in the bloodstream results from sky-high glucose levels, stemming from ingestion of one soft drink, candy bar, or donut on an empty stomach.[5] The average person living in the United States today drinks over 450 sugary 12-ounce soft drinks per year.[6] Each soft drink has ten teaspoons of sugar, so each person consumes more than a quarter-cup of sugar each day just from soft drinks, and a total amount greater than a half-cup from all sources of sugar. As demonstrated in previous and succeeding chapters, that much sugar can suppress the immune system for long periods of time.

Research Links AGEs to Many Age-Related Complications

AGEs can attack virtually every part of the body mimicking a low-grade infection, although a person might not even be aware of it. A lifelong diet high in AGEs leaves the immune system under the constant sway of barely-detectable inflammation. The following are some of the conditions that can be caused by AGEs as we grow older:

- Increased oxidative stress
- Atherosclerosis
- Hypertension[7]
- Cataracts[8]
- Macular degeneration[9]
- Dementia
- Uremia[10]
- Joint stiffness and rheumatoid arthritis[11]
- Kidney damage
- Alzheimer's disease[12]

- Diabetes[13]
- Reduced ability of blood vessels to dilate
- Inflammation
- Increased blood-clotting
- Reduced ability of fats to clear from the bloodstream
- Increased ability of cancer cells to thrive
- Protein damage linked to stiff joints, skin aging, and Alzheimer's and other diseases

"Once formed, the AGE reaction is not reversible, and it gradually accumulates over the lifetime of the protein," observed Dr. Moshe Levi and other kidney specialists writing in a recent issue of the *American Journal of Kidney Diseases.* Dr. Levi said the goal of treatment is to prevent AGEs from forming in the first place.[14] I could not agree more. The goal of every treatment should be prevention.

The glycation process that browns a chicken in the oven is exactly what happens to the proteins in our body. Reacting with sugars, proteins turn brown and fluorescent, lose elasticity, and cross-link to form insoluble masses that generate free radicals. AGEs accumulate in our collagen and skin, cornea, brain, nervous system, arteries, and vital organs as we age. Unfortunately, AGEs are highly resistant to the normal processes of protein turnover and renewal that maintain the healthy tone of youthful body tissues and organs.

As glycation starts, then increases, free radicals form in glycated protein at nearly five times the rate as with non-glycated protein.[16] As a result of this, AGEs and attendant free radicals exert multiple detrimental effects in the body, activating the proinflammatory cytokines that are most common in the elderly. Cytokines have been shown to be particularly high in inflammatory joint diseases (like rheumatoid arthritis), central nervous system disorders (Alzheimer's disease), multiple sclerosis, and ischemia. They have also been shown to promote degeneration of the nerves.

Scientists have known for many years that cooking proteins in the absence of water also forms AGEs. A recent study presented at the annual meeting of the Diabetes Association in San Francisco shows that eating browned foods may cause heart attacks, strokes, and nerve damage. Diabetics suffer a very high incidence of nerve, artery and kidney damage because high blood sugar levels in their bodies markedly accelerate the chemical reactions that form AGEs.

Acrylamide

Reports of the presence of acrylamide, a common AGE, in a variety of fried and oven-cooked foods have caused worldwide concern because this compound has been classified as being probably carcinogenic in humans. Researchers at the University of Redding in the United Kingdom explored variations of the Maillard Reaction and found out that the protein asparagine (common to potatoes and cereals) is the only cause of acrylamide[17].

Moderate levels of acrylamide (5–50 micrograms/kilograms) were measured in heated protein-rich foods and higher levels were found (150–4,000 microg/kg) in carbohydrate-rich foods, such as potato, beetroot, certain heated commercial potato products, and flat breads (pita bread). Acrylamide could not be detected in unheated or boiled foods (<5 microg/kg). Consumption habits indicate that the acrylamide levels in the studied foods could lead to a daily intake of tens of micrograms.[18] The World Health Organization in Geneva, Switzerland, discussed the possible health risk after the announcement by Swedish scientists that acrylamide was present in a wide range of foods, particularly fried, starch-based foods, such as French fries and potato chips.

In a test conducted by the English Food Standards Agency, scientists found a ten-fold difference between normal and overcooked

Vegetarians and AGEs

Vegetarians (plant food, milk products and eggs) and meat eaters were evaluated in a study on AGEs, factoring their general protein consumption, cooking methods, level of food processing, and intake of lysine (a protein) and simple sugars. Two different markers, the less of both the better, were used to test for the number of AGEs in the bloodstream. The vegetarians, eating less protein, including lysine, but four times as much honey, fresh and dried fruit, had higher levels of the two markers than meat eaters. Researchers concluded that the vegetarians ate more simple sugars, like fructose (common to fruits and honey), which exceeds glucose and sucrose (table sugar) in raising the markers.[15] Consumption of excessive sugar is a common risk factor among many vegetarians. If you choose to follow a vegetarian lifestyle, be sure to minimize consumption of such simple sugars, the dangers of which are covered in-depth in my book *Lick the Sugar Habit.*

chips, which experts say is good news, because it means that levels can be limited. But why eat them in the first place? Studies to date show that a minimum temperature of 120°C is needed to start formation of acrylamide in foods, although 140°C to 180°C is optimal. The hotter and longer you bake or fry, the more carcinogens form. The carcinogen tends to attack the thyroid gland, female mammary glands, male testes, and mouth.[19]

Since nerve damage and other inflammatory symptoms are linked to AGEs, caused in part by cooking, how should a person cook? Water inhibits the formation of AGEs, so avoid baking, roasting, and broiling. Boiling and steaming are sensible alternatives. Meats can be sauteed but the meat should be cut very thin and cooked quickly with a small amount of oil. According to Dr. Helen Vlassara, the traditionally cooked, slow-roasted turkey leads the list of AGE offenders, above coffee, cola, and chocolate drinks.[20] But there are other reasons than AGEs for not consuming the last three products mentioned.

According to these new findings, brown foods, such as certain cookies, bread crust, basted meats, beans, and even coffee, may increase nerve damage, particularly in diabetics who are unusually susceptible. On the other hand, since steamed vegetables and whole grains and beans cooked in water are cooked at low temperatures, they do not contain significant amounts of AGEs.[21] The final word is not in about acrylamide, and more research needs to be done to understand the full implications of this free radical.

Tobacco

Tobacco is cured under great heat, causing production of AGEs. Researchers examined tobacco and tobacco smoke for the level of AGEs. Results showed that levels of such glycotoxins (glucose becomes toxic) in the bloodstream were significantly higher in smokers than in nonsmokers. Like other AGEs, glycotoxins exhibit a specific fluorescence when cross-linked to proteins, and are cancer-causing products. AGEs can deteriorate blood vessels in similar fashion. Logic suggests that within smokers are similar conditions, contributing to a greater incidence of atherosclerosis and high prevalence of cancer in smokers.[22] It is also possible to get AGEs from the nicotine patch or gum as used by those who try to quit smoking. Research shows that nornicotine, a metabolite of nicotine, can cause abnormal protein glycation leading to AGEs. Researchers also found that nornicotine modified the structure of prednisone, a commonly prescribed steroid with similarities to glucose, suggesting that other drugs might also be vulnerable to alteration due to smoking.[23]

Four main causes of AGEs have been presented here: sugar, overcooked protein, cooking without water, and smoking. Abstinence from all four will deter AGEs. So quit smoking, eat more raw or lightly cooked food, abstain from refined sugar, and reduce fruit intake to a few pieces per day.

FREE RADICAL DAMAGE AND OXIDATIVE STRESS

All aspects of life depend upon the cell's ability to regulate homeostasis, the state of balance explained in Chapter 2. Every day, a variety of external and internal stressors—toxic chemicals, radiation, pollutants, emotional disturbance, junk food, or food allergies—challenge homeostatic cell regulators. Eventually, such stresses can cause an adverse reaction as the body fails to deal with rampant toxicity, inflammation, and free radicals.

A free radical is a molecule that possesses a free electron, which differs from normal molecules that do not possess a free electron.[24] Free radicals can attack cell membranes, interfere with protein synthesis, lower energy levels, prevent muscle building, and wipe out cellular enzymes, creating metabolic waste products. In limited quantities, free radicals do have beneficial functions, such as assisting nerve impulse transmission, hormone synthesis, immunity, energy production, and muscle contraction. Unfortunately, when too many free radicals develop, the body eventually becomes overwhelmed.[25]

Free radicals react quickly and aggressively due to the instability created by the free electron. Free radicals attack unsaturated lipids, proteins, cell membranes, and enzymes; such attacks, in turn, destroy cells. Worst of all, DNA becomes vulnerable to penetration, allowing damage to the "DNA blueprint" which will be replicated as mutations that the body may be powerless to control. Tissue damage and compromised immune systems can result, describing cancer quite effectively.

Free radicals and antioxidants are mutually opposing chemicals that bind together, canceling each other out. The body checkmates free radicals with antioxidants, free-radical scavenging enzymes, and other free-radical inactivators. Too much toxicity creates free radicals that may overwhelm these defenses, however. This state of affairs is called oxidative stress.[26] Free radical-defeating enzymes depend on the mineral zinc for proper functioning. Zinc levels suffer greatly when the body is out of homeostasis and research shows that ingesting more zinc does not truly affect the problem.[27] I can not stress enough the importance of staying in homeostasis to protect mineral balances and enzyme function.

Sources of Free Radicals

Avoiding free radical sources may seem like an easy task, but they are everywhere. Becoming aware of them is therefore an important step you must take if you are to successfully protect yourself from them. How many factors on the following list are part of your daily life?

General Factors
Aging
Normal Metabolism
Stress

Dietary Factors
Additives
Alcohol—excessive amounts
Coffee
AGE-laden, cooked foods (See pages 39–44.)
Herbicides
Hydrogenated vegetable oils
Pesticides
Sugar in all its many forms—read your labels

Chemical Factors
Air pollutants: asbestos, benzene, carbon monoxide, chlorine, formaldehyde, ozone, and tobacco smoke.
Chemical solvents: cleaning products, glue, paints, paint thinner, medications, perfumes, pesticides, and water pollutants such as chloroform and other trihalomethanes caused by chlorination.

Radiation
Cosmic radiation
Electromagnetic fields
Medical and dental x-rays

Minimizing Free Radicals

Physical and emotional stress can contribute to oxidative stress, most notably through the release of cortisol, an anti-inflammatory adrenal hormone. Cortisol suppresses the immune system and forms free radicals. Athletes experience this process in the wake of intense workouts that stress the body. The following list contains tips for minimizing free radicals.

- Choose organic, pesticide-free, additive-free foods.

- Eat as little sugar as possible.

- Drink purified water.

- Avoid exposure to volatile chemicals, including perfume, hair spray, glue, paint, gasoline, solvents, and smoke.

- Limit exposure to air pollution: keep your windows closed when driving in heavy traffic, and stay off busy streets when exercising.

- When outdoors, limit the amount of time you spend in direct sunlight, especially at midday.

- Check your house for radon gas. (Hardware and home supply stores sell inexpensive testing kits; for more information, see www.radonzone.com.)

- Get medical and dental x-rays only when absolutely necessary.

- Take medications only when your doctor requires it. (Note: Always consult your doctor before you stop taking any medicine that he or she has prescribed.)

Illnesses Associated with Oxidative Stress

Whatever the cause of oxidative stress, prevention is key, or diseases from the following list can strike.

Gastrointestinal tract: pancreatitis, liver damage, and leaky gut syndrome.

Brain and nervous system: Parkinson's disease, Alzheimer's disease, hypertension, and/or multiple sclerosis.

Heart and blood vessels: atherosclerosis and/or coronary thrombosis.

Lungs: asthma, emphysema and/or chronic pulmonary disease.

Eyes: cataracts, retinopathy, and macular degeneration.

Joints: rheumatoid arthritis.

Kidneys: glomerulonephritis (inflammation of the kidney).

Skin: wrinkles.

Body in general: accelerated aging, cancer, autoimmune diseases, inflammatory states, AIDS, lupus, diabetes.

Determining Oxidative Stress

The body excretes various by-products of oxidative stress, oxidized DNA bases, lipid peroxides, and malonidialhyde from damaged lipids and proteins in the urine. It is possible to test for these factors. High levels probably indicate a greater chance of acquiring an oxidative stress-related disease, or the aggravation and acceleration of an existing one. As an example of the latter, people with Down syndrome suffer enormous oxidative stress from over-production of hydrogen peroxide, a potent oxidizer. They frequently develop Alzheimer's-like symptoms in their 30s.[28] Go through the list of causes of oxidative stress again and see what you can comfortably eliminate from your life. The less stressors your body is exposed to, the more it will be able to maintain a healthy homeostasis.

PSYCHOLOGICAL STRESS
(Body-Mind Connection, Brain Allergies, Emotional Difficulties, Psychic Stress, Psycho-neuro-gastro-endrocrino-immunology, and Psychoneuroimmunology)

What and how a person thinks and feels can affect his or her digestion. Conversely, if a food does not digest properly, it can affect how a person thinks and feels. Problems can develop either way. This mind-body connection has been given a long medical name: psychoneuroimmunology. Considering information presented in sections of this book, a better but even more tongue-twisting name is *psycho-neuro-gastro-endrocrino-immunology*. "Endocrino" relates to endocrine glands secreting hormones into the bloodstream that regulate homeostasis and should be added to the word. Another addition should be "gastro" because of the gastrointestinal tract's primary function of digesting foods. Failure to properly digest causes food particles to be released into the bloodstream, becoming an allergy looking for a target—the brain being one of them.

In the previous chapter, a list of symptoms for allergies with body-wide effects was presented. The list on the following page details ailments that specifically affect the brain.

How Digestion Affects the Mind

In Chapter 2, we presented information about our body chemistry and homeostasis. As we saw, when minerals become depleted, they exhaust certain mineral-dependent enzymes. This, in turn, hampers food digestion, allowing food particles into the bloodstream. The food particles cause the immune system to respond, and inflammation is one of the responses. The brain is just as susceptible to these allergens and inflammation as the rest of the body, creating great havoc between the ears.[32]

Dr. T. C. Theoharides says, "mast cells can participate in the regulation of blood-brain permeability." It has been stated that mast cells become activated in food allergy. Thus, food allergens can cause significant, localized, increased permeability in the blood-brain barrier. Theoharides goes on to say that this allergy and consequent inflammation can affect the brain, and, depending on the part, can produce notable changes in the person's thoughts and actions.[33]

Symptoms of Brain Allergy

Aggression	Daydreaming	Math, spelling, and
Anger for no	Emotionally	reading errors
apparent reason	sensitive	Memory loss
Anxiety	Erratic	Mood swings
Attention deficit	Fearful	Morbid
disorder (ADD)	Hallucinations	Not open to
Changes in	Hearing without	reason
handwriting	comprehension	Nightmares
Chews clothes	Hyperactivity,	Panic attacks
and bedclothes	including	Paranoia
Clumsiness	fidgeting	Phobias
Compulsive	Impatience	Poor self-image
behavior	Inability to be	Poor work habits
Confusion,	pleased	Restlessness
disorientation,	Indecisive	Screaming attacks
brain fogging,	Indifference to work,	Slow metabolism
and blankness	clothes, hygiene,	Slurred, stammering,
Delusions	friends, etc.	and stuttering
Depression	Irresponsibility	speech
Detached or unreal	Irritability	Suicidal feelings
feeling	Lethargy (mental	Sulky
Difficulty waking up	and physical)	Tenseness
Dyslexia and other	Loss of sex drive	Uncooperative
learning disabilities	(low libido)	Weepiness [29,30,31]

Dr. Rothenberg believes that food allergies most profoundly affect the limbic region of the brain. This brain area and its associated emotions, memories, and autonomic functions—including body temperature, sexuality, blood pressure, sleep, hunger, and thirst—can be greatly impacted by allergies.[34] In addition, these food allergies act as false kinins, causing inflammation, and interfere with brain function and behavior by interrupting neurotransmitter (messenger chemicals that work throughout the body) pathways.[35]

Dr. Philpott writes in *Brain Allergies*, "If the part of the brain affected is one that controls certain behavioral patterns, this allergic irritation will produce recognizable mental and/or behavior changes."[36] A person can become manic, depressed, autistic, delusional, bipolar, wildly excited, or be totally apathetic.[37] Food addictions change the level of neurotransmitters in the brain, affecting all behavior patterns. They can also swell brain tissues, irritating sensitive nerves to cause great emotional turmoil.[38] Chemical allergies can cause similar problems as food which passes the blood-brain barrier.

During an allergic reaction, the body leaks histamine from the capillaries, causing swelling around them. Dr. Marshall Mandell, author of *Dr. Mandell's 5 Day Allergy Relief System,* believes that the same reaction takes place in brain cells when you eat an allergen-inducing food. Additionally, Dr. Mandell proposes that spasms in small brain arteries reduce the flow of glucose, oxygen, and other nutrients—a process similar to the constricted bronchiole tubes associated with asthma attacks. Whether a histamine reaction or an arterial spasm, mood and behavior changes would naturally result, usually leading to depression, which may explain why some people feel great when they fast.[39] During a fast, the foods that cause the emotional problems have been removed and many negative feelings disappear.

Dr. Mandell found that 92.2 percent of hospitalized schizophrenic patients were allergic to one or more common food substances. Testing a group of patients diagnosed as hard-to-treat neurotics, he found 88 percent were allergic to wheat, 50 percent to corn, and 60 percent to milk. He theorized that faulty digestion results in undigested protein pieces that mimic kinins when absorbed, creating harmful reactions. Dr. Philpott takes a different view, believing that these particles actually cause kinin-mediated inflammation.[40] It does not matter which doctor is right: inflammation is the end result either way. Another study revealed that during ragweed seasons, allergic patients reported higher levels of physical and mental fatigue, sadness, reduced motivation, and less pleasure. The head researcher, Dr. P. Marshall, suggests that allergic reactions create biochemical changes that directly affect the central nervous system and mood.[41]

I read this letter on the web and thought many of you would identify with it:

For the past 3 weeks, I have been an awful person to deal with at work and at home! I am allergic mainly to dust and mold and this time (September) every year I suffer from severe allergies. I just started getting allergy shots a few months ago, and I go every week faithfully! I also take Zyrtec every morning, and I use nasal spray every day. All of this still does not take away my suffering at this time of the year! I thought I was nuts with the moods I was having. Now, I just have to get my fiancé to believe that it is my allergies that yell at him and not me (ha ha)!

If this woman would just find and remove foods to which she reacts, she would not have to get her fiancé to believe anything. Philpott believes that 70 to 80 percent of people with mental disorders have reactions to food. Dr. Theron Randolph, in his well-recognized book, *Clinical Ecology,* stated his belief that more than half of the so-called psychosomatic reactions are in reality undiagnosed allergic reactions.[42] Again we turn to Hippocrates who understood, many centuries ago, how food can affect the brain.

And thus, also, if one who has been accustomed to dine, and this rule agrees with him, should not dine at the accustomed hour, he will straightway feel great loss of strength, trembling, and want of spirits; the eyes of such a person will become more pallid, his urine thick and hot, his mouth bitter; his bowels will seem, as it were, to hang loose; he will suffer from vertigo, lowness of spirit, and inactivity . . . If he should attempt to take at supper the same food which he was wont to partake of at dinner . . . these things, passing downwards, with tormina (achy, colicky pain) and rumbling, burn up his bowels; he experiences insomnolency (unnatural sleep) or troubled and disturbed dreams; and to many of them these symptoms are the commencement of some disease.

Hippocrates described a disorder with many symptoms. He was aware of the fascinating phenomena of addiction to the allergenic food, marked by withdrawal symptoms if the food is not eaten regularly. This withdrawal phenomenon has been typically misconstrued as a hypoglycemic reaction. Frequent cravings for allergenic foods and marked withdrawal discomforts make investigation and treatment of food allergy a complicated business.[43]

How the Mind Affects the Body and Digestion

Not only does the body's reaction to the environment affect the brain, the reverse is also true.[44] Prolonged psychological stress that includes competition, goal-oriented behavior, time pressures, or anger or any other negative emotion, can cause problems as well. Stomach acid output may increase or decrease, interfering with pancreatic enzymes that break down foods in the small intestine. Poor digestive enzyme activity results in food particles that act as allergens, kinin mimics, and neurotransmitter substitutes, an overload of which causes inflammation and taxes the immune system.[45]

Depression, with its crippling symptoms of hopelessness, apathy, appetite disorder, irritability, sadness, and low energy, seems to predispose individuals to a wide range of allergens.[46] Triggered by life changes like divorce, unemployment, grief, early childhood trauma, or, most insidiously, no clear cause, depression can cause food allergies. Understanding and dealing with past traumas can be essential to a person's recovery from food allergies, though abstinence from reactive foods for some time may still be necessary. Dr. Paul Black's research shows that the brain is likely to be involved in immune system regulation. Stress, psychological or physical, launches cytokines that may contribute to the beginning of inflammatory diseases, activating mast cells, releasing neuropeptides (neurotransmitter with direct effect on the nervous system), and stress hormones such as catecholamines, corticosteroids, growth hormone, and glucagons.[47] Chronic stress suppresses immune function with a vicious double-whammy, first by creating more vulnerability to disease and secondly by impairing the body's anti-inflammatory processes. Glucocorticoid, a hormone that stops inflammation when the threat is over, reacts badly in a high-stress environment, allowing cytokines to go unchecked.

Examining the relationship between ongoing stress and disease, researchers from Washington University compared twenty-five parents of children undergoing cancer treatment to twenty-five parents of healthy children. Mental health, effects of social support, and immune system responses were measured. Parents of cancer patients reported more psychological distress than parents with healthy children and were found to have diminished glucocorticoid sensitivity. However, researchers also found that social support lessened the immunologic consequences of caring for a child with cancer. Gregory E. Miller, PhD, from Washington University, says, "These findings suggest a mechanism through which psychological stress could influence the onset and/or progression of conditions that involve excessive inflammation, like allergic, autoimmune, cardiovascular, infectious, and rheumatologic illnesses. Inflammation can affect any tissue or any organ in the body." Dr. Miller feels that anxiety, upsetting thoughts, feelings of helplessness, and lack of sleep can trigger this mechanism.[48]

Emory University researchers found that stress and depression influence the outcomes in immune-related disorders, including cancer and infectious diseases. Evidence suggests that an inflammatory immune response from any source can cause behavioral symptoms that are similar to chronic stress or major depression.[49]

Free Radicals and Oxidative Stress

Distress takes hold in many situations. A group of researchers investigated young volunteers who were exposed to political intolerance, awareness of potential military attacks, permanent stand-by-duty, and reduced holidays. These researchers also studied stress consisting of everyday mortal danger in military actions lasting more than three months. Similarly, both study groups exhibited free radicals leading to oxidative stress as assessed by increased plasma superoxide and malondialdehyde, and a decrease in antioxidants. It is important to find ways to relieve the feelings of stress, as these feelings can be another stressor and overload the body's homeostatic mechanisms. Do not make the stressful feeling become distressful. When under heavy psychological stress make sure you eat correctly, sleep well, and exercise.[50]

The Pairing of Allergies and Emotions

Whether allergies cause emotional problems, or the reverse, the compulsive eater knows he or she must eat a certain food to relieve or prevent mental sluggishness, irritability, fatigue, weakness, headaches, or other brain allergy symptoms.[51] Since anything that throws the body out of homeostasis, whether physical or mental, can cause inflammation and disease, all factors must be dealt with at the same time. Which comes first, emotional problems or allergies? The answer to this question is not as important as finding a way to alleviate both of them. This can be achieved by eliminating the foods to which you are allergic or sensitive, and by ensuring that the stress in your life does not become distress.

PART TWO

Inflammation and Disease

5

Health Conditions
Caused by or Associated
With Inflammation

This section of the book will show how inflammation is related to many diseases. I have written about only those diseases that I have been able to document with medical research. However, I believe that in the future there will be many more diseases for which inflammation will be verified as playing a role. Eventually, I think research will probably reveal that inflammation either causes or is associated with most diseases.

Despite the importance of screening for inflammation to ensure good health, many doctors and patients alike still fail to consider inflammation's role in the disease process. This is unfortunate, since many conventionally regarded symptoms are actually in themselves symptoms of a deeper, underlying cause—chronic inflammation. Although the inflammatory response is similar in all diseases it is associated with, the causes can be diverse. Unless the conditions that are causing the chronic inflammatory response are properly dealt with, lasting relief is not possible. Conversely, when inflammation is reversed, your remaining symptoms will usually resolve themselves, as well. In the pages that follow, I discuss the disease conditions most commonly associated with inflammation, and show you what to consider if you suffer from them. By addressing the factors that can lead to inflammation, you will significantly improve your ability to maintain your health and to recover from most diseases.

ALZHEIMER'S DISEASE

Alzheimer's disease (AD) is one of several disorders that cause the gradual loss of brain cells, leading to mental deterioration. The disease was first described in 1906 by German physician, Dr. Alois Alzheimer. Although the disease was once considered rare, research has shown that today it is the leading cause of dementia (loss of mental functions).

In AD, plaque builds up and causes inflammation in the neurons of the brain.[1] This inflammatory cascade involves cytokines and prostaglandins. As this process continues, it accelerates the loss of neurons. Studies show that cytokines create the plaques. "Inflammation is directly damaging neurons," said Dr. Paul Aisen, a professor of neurology at Georgetown University Medical Center.[2] The body produces antibodies to control the inflammation, but antibodies can only do so much. Eventually the body becomes overwhelmed by inflammation that persists, and is unable to stop it.[3]

Oxidative stress results in metal accumulations, cell damage, and formations of AGEs. Researchers claim that oxidative stress is the element that links changes seen in patients with AD. A reduction of oxidative stress will have a dramatic effect on reducing the incidence or progression of the disease.[4] Dr. D.A. Butterfield and associates found that AD could be induced by AGEs.[5] Therefore, AGEs can influence the beginnings as well as the progression of the condition.

Animal studies also show that foods with strong antioxidant properties, such as blueberries, freeze-dried spinach, and spices like turmeric, reduce physical complications caused by AD.[6] Make sure you are not allergic to any one of them. The Body Monitor Kit will help you test for allergies (see page 128). Dr. M.M. Verbeek, from the Netherlands, states in a journal article, "There is an increasing amount of evidence that the formation of senile plaques is accompanied by an acute phase reaction, involving the production of several inflammation-associated proteins."[7] He does not state what the acute phase reaction is, but it certainly could be a food allergy.

Scientists have shown that trace amounts of mercury can cause nerve damage similar to AD. The level of mercury exposure used in the test was well below those levels found in many humans with mercury/silver amalgam dental fillings. The research has shown that Alzheimer's patients have at least three times higher blood levels of mercury compared to controls.[8] There are blood tests to test for mercury toxicity. (See Chapter 8.)

Another metal can also be a problem in AD. Excessive iron accumulation in the brain is a pattern consistent with the disease. A simple blood test can be used to evaluate the level of iron in the blood.[9] If iron levels are excessive, steps should be taken to reduce them.

People who exercised vigorously at least three times per week were considered highly active and had the lowest Alzheimer's risk. Even those who engaged in light or moderate exercise also saw significant reductions in their risks for AD and mental decline.[10] Dr. R. P. Friedland and associates found that diversity of activity and intensity of intellectual activities were reduced in patients with AD as compared to normal people. They could not tell whether inactivity lead to the disease, if inactivity was an effect of the disease, or if it was both.[11] It seems logical not to worry about what caused the inactivity. It makes more sense to finish this book because this is certainly an intellectual activity. When you are finished reading this chapter, go get some exercise, and do not forget to do both of these activities every day.

BLOOD SUGAR PROBLEMS

Diabetes Mellitus (high blood sugar), Hypoglycemia (low blood sugar), and Metabolic Syndrome

Three classes of blood sugar ailments concern us here: hypoglycemia, diabetes, and metabolic syndrome. They relate to each other because in all cases glucose does not assimilate into the body properly. Diabetes, the fastest growing disease in the United States, as well as the rest of the world, is the fifth-leading killer in the United States. Diagnosed cases in America run to about one in fourteen or 7.3 percent of the population, but when undiagnosed cases are factored in, a one in ten rate becomes possible.[1]

Diabetes is a group of serious diseases characterized by high blood sugar levels that result from defects in the body's ability to produce and/or use insulin. These problems can lead to severely debilitating or fatal complications, such as coronary heart disease, atherosclerosis, stroke, blindness, kidney disease, amputations, and periodontal disease. They can also result in a higher incidence of infections.

Diabetes has two classes: Type I (child-onset) and Type II (adult-onset). Type I diabetics have malfunctioning Islets of Langerhans in the pancreas and suffer from a lack of insulin. Type II diabetics produce sufficient insulin, but the insulin is unable to get into the cells to perform its function. Over 90 percent of diabetics are adult-onset.

Type I Diabetes

Introduction of cow milk formulas in infancy may increase the risk of Type I diabetes. Cow milk, like sugar, can increase the permeability of the GI tract wall, leading to partially digested foods in the bloodstream, a precursor to inflammation and diseases.[2] A group of researchers at Medical College of Wisconsin recommend that children with insulin-dependent diabetes mellitus (IDDM) be tested for celiac disease (gluten intolerance). I feel these children should also be tested for all allergies. Any food or chemical that is frequently eaten or encountered has the potential of becoming an allergen or addictive, radically altering sugar levels and causing diabetes.[3]

Type II Diabetes

Type II diabetes is considered an autoimmune disease. The body produces auto-antibodies to its own T-cells. The T-cells help create lesions that lead to inflammation and cell deterioration.[4] I believe that autoimmune diseases are caused by environmental triggers which lead to a malfunctioning in the body. I do not believe the body turns against itself without good reason.

Researchers say that several inflammation markers increase in people who have diabetes. Dr. Bruce Duncan studied more than 10,000 people for nine years, none of whom had diabetes at the beginning of the study. In the follow-up, Dr. Duncan and his colleagues found an association between higher levels of inflammatory markers and the onset of Type II diabetes. He says, "Higher levels of these markers led to two to three times the risk of developing diabetes."[5]

Philpott shows that the ultimate effect of continual allergic exposure is the degradation of pancreatic function, leading to diabetes. Undigested food particles (allergens) get into the bloodstream and a vicious cycle ensues. Chronic inflammation produced by allergens and other irritants provokes a continual excess of endorphins. This eventually decreases the ability of the pancreas to produce bicarbonate, which is needed to neutralize hydrochloric acid that saturates food. Without bicarbonate, the small intestines become acidic, inhibiting the production of proteolytic enzymes produced by the pancreas, further complicating the process of food digestion.[6] The mechanism is not clear, but let me give you an example. If a person is allergic to eggs (which have no simple sugar to raise blood glucose), the blood glucose can flair up. This does not happen to everyone who is allergic to eggs, but it is a little-known phenomenon that can happen with any food.[7]

Philpott also studied the effect of allergic reactions on blood sugar levels and found that any food allergen could raise glucose levels above normal. It was not just carbohydrates that did this, but also proteins and/or fats.[8] While a person may not eat simple sugars in excess, a given food might still react and abnormally raise blood glucose levels if eaten on a consistent basis, thus facilitating diabetes.

Dr A.D. Pradhan found that elevated CRP and interleukin are also associated with a higher-than-average risk of developing Type II diabetes.[9] Over a period of years, disease-free women's CRP and interleukin levels were studied. It was found that those with elevated levels throughout the years were the ones more likely to develop diabetes. Inflammation may signal potentially dangerous metabolic imbalances that fuel central obesity and insulin resistance.[10] Trying to prevent inflammation from destroying insulin-producing cells occupies much research time.[11] It would seem wiser to find out what causes inflammation.

Excess body fat, especially around the mid-section, a major risk factor for diabetes, may also be part of the inflammatory picture. Fat cells produce cytokines, the proteins that promote inflammation. Studies have shown that people who develop Type II diabetes have relatively high levels of these cytokines. Researchers think the cytokines may interfere with the body's ability to use its own insulin, thus bringing on diabetes.

In Type II diabetes, oxidative damage has been implicated in both the development of the disease and its many complications. Free radicals inhibit glucose metabolism, thereby causing an overload of sugar in the blood. Increased blood sugar levels, in turn, also cause AGEs.[12] As has been stated (see Chapter 4), AGEs form toxic compounds when sugar, proteins, and fat are cooked at high temperatures for long periods of time. These compounds may cause inflammation and increase blood vessel damage in diabetics.[13] Other factors that promote inflammation and diabetes are obesity, smoking, and hypertension.[14]

It is wise for diabetics to eat raw, boiled, or steamed food. It is also important for diabetics to keep their blood sugar in the normal range as much as possible so that the excess sugar in the bloodstream will not form AGEs. Check to see if any foods that you regularly eat elevate blood sugar, and if so remove them from your diet. My Food Plan III (see Chapter 7) eliminates most of these problems. It is wise to not smoke, maintain normal weight, and deal with the stress in your life to keep your blood pressure in the normal range.

Hypoglycemia

Hypoglycemia (low blood sugar) is frequently caused by excess sugar in the diet, food allergy, and obesity.[15] A healthy body is able to metabolize two teaspoons of sugar easily. An unhealthy body is not able to tolerate sugar at all. If you eat sugar, or foods that are easily converted to sugar by the body, the sharp rise in blood sugar causes too great an increase in the levels of insulin, as well as upsets mineral relationships. Sugar can also suppress the immune system. In addition, the increase in insulin can result in the blood sugar being driven too low, too fast. Starches like potatoes, beans, carrots, and rice are also converted to simple sugars rapidly if eaten alone, but if eaten with protein and fat, as found in Food Plan III on page 133, will not raise glucose and insulin levels above normal and are healthy foods.

Since the brain does not store a great deal of sugar, like the muscles do, it is very sensitive to the levels of blood sugar. If the brain does not get the correct amount of sugar it needs to operate properly, various symptoms can occur. When this is done over and over, the pancreas can malfunction, as well. (The pancreas can malfunction when the brain is operating properly too, of course.) Philpott discovered that an allergenic food can provoke not only diabetes or high blood sugar, but also hypoglycemia. Both foods and chemicals that are allergenic to a person can decrease or increase sugar levels.

Metabolic Syndrome

Metabolic syndrome is also known as Metabolic Syndrome X, Syndrome X, Insulin Resistance Syndrome, and Reduced Insulin Sensitivity. It is a cluster of metabolic abnormalities, including insulin resistance, high blood glucose, high blood pressure, low high density lipoprotein (HDL), high cholesterol, and high triglycerides. Either overall obesity or mid-section obesity can be present, but central obesity is more prevalent. Many of these factors by themselves can cause inflammation, adversely affecting glycemic control. In addition, hyperinsulinemia/insulin resistance can increase inflammation.[16] The majority of individuals who die from cardiovascular disease show unhealthy levels in two or more metabolic abnormalities.[17]

A national survey suggests that metabolic syndrome affects about 24 percent of adults who are twenty to seventy years of age. These statistics may become larger as the population ages and continues to increase in weight. People with the syndrome are about twice as likely to develop heart disease, and over four times as likely to develop Type II diabetes, compared with subjects who do not have metabolic syndrome. This close association of Type II diabetes and heart disease suggests that there is a common denominator in both diseases. That common denominator might be insulin resistance.[18] Blood tests showing fasting insulin and triglycerides provide a simple means of screening for insulin resistance in the general population.[19]

A large, generally male, segment of the adult population of industrialized countries develops metabolic syndrome. Causes include hormonal and lifestyle factors such as obesity, physical inactivity, overeating, and eating sugar and other simple carbohydrates excessively.[20] One medical journal that I read summed up the problem by saying the following: "Diet and lifestyle are effective strategies, but they must compete with behaviors that have instant gratification. Our society has turned its focus away from the long-term rewards of good sustainable behaviors and has instead focused on short-term rewards of unsustainable behaviors. To tame the behaviors that promote the metabolic syndrome, simple answers from diet and drug therapy will require support from society to be effective."[21]

Unfortunately, fast foods, antibiotics and other drugs, computers, and other twenty-first century lifestyle factors give instant gratification. Changing habits, natural healing, and fighting food allergies takes more time and effort than most people are willing to devote to their health.

What to Do

In looking to stop the cause of blood sugar problems, it is necessary to consider a variety of lifestyle adjustments. These include:

• Obtaining and maintaining normal weight. Being overweight is the most obvious sign that you are not eating correctly.

• Eating no foods containing simple sugar or caffeine, as caffeine triggers the liver to release stored sugar into the bloodstream. Food Plan III on page 133 is best.

• Checking for food allergies, with an emphasis on dairy products and gluten.

• Eating many healthy, small meals a day. Each person is different, but some people need to eat every hour, while others need to eat only every two hours. It is best to have a little protein, fat, and complex carbohydrate for each snack.

• Checking for low-grade infection, causing inflammation.

• Making sure that the stress in your life does not become distress.

These suggestions are good for fighting all forms of sugar problems and insulin resistance.

CANCER

The concept that inflammation causes cancer has been around for more than a century. The scientists Julius Vogel (1814–1880) and Rudolph Virchow (1812–1902) put forth the theory that the growth of cancer was due to irritation. Both thought that irritation caused inflammation and excessive cellular growth. This theory continued into the twentieth century, although it was superseded by sophisticated genetic explanations.[1]

Recently, some British scientists have concluded that the long-term over-activation of the immune system (such as through irritation or infection, which are sources of inflammation) may be the single most important cause of cancer. They call any inflamed tissue "a melting pot of cancer-causing molecules." "The long-standing over-activation of the immune system is the key event in the genesis of many forms of the disease," says Dr. Angus Dalgleish of the Department of Oncology, University of Leicester. "My research shows that there is an elevation of CRP in most cancers: breast, lung, colorectal, prostate, and pancreatic cancer."[2]

Other researchers have also identified inflammation as a significant factor in the development of solid tumor malignancies. There are chronic inflammatory conditions that do not have an established cause, infections being ruled out. This strongly suggests that the process of inflammation provides the prerequisite environment for the development of malignancy.[3]

"Tumors when they're developing are just proliferating cells. The theory is that it looks much like a wound to the host. So inflammatory cells come in and do their job. They urge the growth onward," said Dr. Lisa Coussens, from the department of pathology and Cancer Research Institute at the University of California at San Francisco.[4]

Chronic pancreatitis is inflammation of the pancreas. It is associated with an increased risk of developing pancreatic cancer. Chromosome damage and cellular proliferation, both of which relate to inflammation, can change pancreatic cells into malignancies. Cytokines and free radicals can increase the number of cells, and impede the body's natural tumor defenses. Researchers at the Hopkins Kimmel Cancer Center have also found that the earliest stages of prostate cancer may develop from lesions generally associated with chronic inflammation. Dr. Emilio Williams, head researcher in the study, believes that these irritations progress to pre-cancerous lesions, and are strongly linked to cancer.

Why does a person develop these lesions in the first place? The following are among the primary reasons that such pre-cancerous conditions are established.

Chronic Infections

Chronic inflammation caused by infections increases the risk of certain human cancers, including those of the liver (hepatitis B virus), cervix (human papilloma virus), stomach (*helicobacter pylori*), and bladder (schistosomiasis). These infections may contribute to the development of cancer.[5] But not all inflammatory conditions are infection related. Read on for more causes.

Free Radical Damage and Oxidative Stress

The research of Dr. E. Hietanen shows that oxidative stress may be associated with malignant diseases of all types.[6] Free radicals attack many cellular targets including membranes, proteins, and nucleic acids, and cause structural damage to DNA.[7] Three markers of free radicals were studied in cancer patients. These markers are:

- Level of lipid peroxidation products (MDA level) in the plasma.

- The activity of erythrocyte antioxidant defense enzymes that defend against free radicals.

- Superoxide dismutase (SOD) and catalase (CAT), enzymes that protect us against free radicals.

Each of these markers were significantly higher in patients with early and advanced cancers in comparison to the healthy volunteers.[8]

Stress

Years ago I read about research professors, one at Stanford University and the other at the University of California at Berkeley, who thought that psychological factors did not play a role in cancer. To prove this, the professors enlisted fifty women who had breast cancer. These patients, of similar age and socio-economic background, were divided into two groups. One group was asked to attend group therapy once a week, while the other group was not asked to change their routine in any way.

In group therapy sessions, the therapist told the cancer patients to take charge of their life, finances, children, home, and cancer. No diets were changed. The outcome in this research showed that the people in the therapy group lived about two years longer than the group who had not attended therapy. The professors found that their previous beliefs were incorrect, realizing that psychological factors did indeed play a role in cancer. I feel that if the diet had been changed, as well, the added years in the therapy group would have been extended.

I remember reading another research paper showing the roles that stress and smoking play in the cancer process. Half of the volunteers had cancer and half did not, but all of them smoked. A questionnaire to each participant showed that both groups had the same problems with children, spouses, work, and money. The difference was the people who had cancer had a tragic outlook on life. The stress of life had become distress to these people, and had made a difference in the development of their cancer. Both stress and smoking cause inflammation, so these smoking cancer patients had two conditions that were detrimental to their health. It is not life's situations, but how we deal with them, that can cause the distress and disease.

AGEs

Dr. Y. Yamamoto found that AGEs plays an active role in pancreatic cancer.[9] Dr. Hiroki Kuniyasu also established that AGEs are closely associated with early and advanced stages of gastric cancer.[10] It would be wise to be on Food Plan III on page 133 if you are dealing with pancreatitis, pancreatic cancer, or gastric cancer. Not only will you get a minimum of AGEs, but many other cancer-causing agents will also be eliminated from your diet.

Food Allergy

In 1971, Dr. William McWhorter investigated 6,108 adults during the First National Health and Nutrition Examination Survey. His objective was to focus on the relationship between a history of allergy and the subsequent risk of developing cancer. The group with allergies constituted 30 percent of the sample. He found that allergy sufferers—controlled for race, sex, age, and smoking history—had a "highly significant positive association between history of allergy and development of cancer." A family history of allergy was also a risk factor for subsequent cancer.[11]

In his book, *Nutrition in Health and Disease,* Dr. Maurice Shils supports McWhorter's findings in one significant area. Three separate studies reviewed by Shils found a very high incidence of intestinal lymphomas in celiac patients: 10 percent in one study, 6.2 percent in a second, and 6.9 percent in a third. Males above forty years of age, with long-standing celiac disease who are not eating a gluten-free diet, are a major risk group.[12] People who have lymphomas should all be tested for food allergy. Lymphoma occurs when the body produces too many of a certain type of cells, known as B-cells, which are capable of causing cancer tumors.

Another study shows the relationship of non-Hodgkin's lymphoma, a cancer of the immune system, and food allergy. This overproduction of cells leading to such cancer is prompted when certain components of the immune system are inactivated.[13] Other factors that put people at risk for non-Hodgkin's lymphoma are a history of splenectomy (surgical removal of spleen), gonorrhea, and polio in men and endocrine gland disorders in women. Obesity was also seen as a risk factor.[14]

Since it is known that food allergy, AGEs, free radicals, or other foreign invaders suppress the immune system and cause inflammation, it would be wise for cancer patients to minimize all forms of antigens by following Food Plan III on page 133. The immune system needs to be as healthy as possible to deal with the cancer. A detoxification program is also called for. (See Chapter 8.)

CANDIDA ALBICANS

Candida, Candidiasis, Systemic Candidiasis, Thrush

Candida albicans is a yeast organism that lives in all of our bodies, but seems to overgrow in more and more women and men today. It is a normal flora in our bodies, a simple form of yeast. When we have a balanced body chemistry and a strong immune system, it lives happily within us, but when we upset our minerals and have a low concentration of functioning calcium, our immune system cannot keep *Candida* in balance and it overgrows. When this occurs, *Candida* can colonize the mouth, vagina or intestinal tract and migrates to other parts and organs of the body. In the mouth or vagina it is known as thrush. In the intestinal tract it is known as candidiasis.

Candida can develop a fungus-like structure that is capable of burrowing roots into the intestinal walls. A leaky or over-permeable intestine can result in undigested food particles coming more easily into contact with the bloodstream, and thus further inflammation. Toxins are also more easily absorbed into the blood from a leaky, over-permeable gut, resulting in increased stress on the liver, which is already overburdened with *Candida* toxins. As liver detoxifying enzymes become overloaded due to this process, sensitivity to odors, environmental factors, and natural chemicals in many foods can develop, producing varied symptoms and often a severely debilitating fatigue.[1]

Candida overgrowth can cause an individual to become sensitized not only to *Candida* but also to other yeasts. The presence of *Candida* in the intestines then causes chronic allergic reactions like bloating and inflammation. The consumption of yeast in the diet, from bread, wine, beer, stock cubes and yeast extract, can aggravate these symptoms or cause additional allergic reactions.

Causes of *Candida* Overgrowth

Candidaisis is most often attributed to one or more of the following:

- Alcohol
- Antacids and anti-ulcer medications
- Antibiotics
- Birth control pills/oral contraceptives
- Chemicals and toxins
- Chemotherapy
- Chronic constipation or diarrhea
- Diabetes
- Diets high in sugar
- Excessive stress
- Having a repressed immune system due to medication or disease
- Intestinal parasites
- Multiple pregnancies
- Steroids
- Thyroid disease

Symptoms

Candida overgrowth can cause a wide variety of symptoms. Many times the symptoms are similar to allergies because *Candida* can cause or mimic allergies. Often people may experience as many as twenty of the following list of symptoms.

Allergic and Upper Respiratory

- Blurred vision
- Body aches and tension
- Bronchitis (recurrent)
- Burning or tingling
- Headaches
- Head/neck tension
- Nasal congestion
- Numbness

- Chemical sensitivity
- Chest pain
- Coughing
- Earaches
- Hay fever (allergic rhinitis)
- Painful, swollen, stiff joints

- Shortness of breath
- Sinusitis
- Sore throats
- Swollen lips or face
- Urticaria (hives, wheals or welts)

Cognitive

- Attention deficit disorder
- ADHD
- Confusion
- Disorientation
- Drowsiness
- Fatigue

- Feelings of unreality
- Hyperactivity
- Inability to concentrate
- Obsessive-compulsive disorder
- Poor memory

Emotional

- Anxiety
- Depression
- Irritability

- Mood swings
- Nervousness

Gastrointestinal

- Bloating
- Constipation
- Diarrhea
- Dry mouth
- Gas
- Halitosis (bad breath)
- Heartburn

- Indigestion
- Inflammation
- Irritable bowel syndrome (IBS)
- Lactose intolerance
- Oral thrush
- Rectal itch

Genitourinary

- Bladder infection (recurrent)
- Burning on urination
- Cystitis (inflammation of the bladder)
- Fluid retention (edema)
- Frequent urination
- Impotency
- Infertility
- Loss of sexual feelings
- Prostitis

Glandular and Autoimmune

- Adrenal and thyroid gland malfunction
- Cold hands or feet
- Diabetes mellitus
- Hypoglycemia
- Hypothyroidism
- Low body temperature
- Lupus

Skin

- Acne
- Athlete's foot
- Dandruff
- Diaper rash
- Dry skin
- Eczema
- Excessive perspiration
- Facial rash
- Fungus infection of the nails
- Impetigo (skin infection)
- Inflammation of hair follicles (candidiasis folliculitis)
- Psoriasis
- Seborrheic dermatitis
- Tinea cruris (jock itch)

Women's Issues

- Cramps
- Endometriosis (irregular, painful menstruation)
- Menstrual irregularities
- Painful intercourse
- Premenstrual syndrome (PMS)
- Recurrent yeast vaginitis
- Vaginal burning, itching or discharge

Other

- Chronic fatigue
- Conjunctivitis
- Eye fatigue
- Excessive weight loss
- Insomnia

- Muscle pain
- Muscle weakness
- Obesity
- Symptoms worse upon waking
- Tingling and numbness[2]

Diagnosis and Treatment

It is difficult to diagnose intestinal candidiasis, since it is normal for most individuals to have some of this yeast harmlessly resident in their digestive tract. Many people can be helped by following a green juice diet for three days, then going on Food Plan III for at least two months. This does not include any sugar, alcohol, fruit, dairy (except butter), wheat, nuts, or seeds. It does include lots of vegetables, some protein, and some fat. Also use lots of raw garlic and onions in your salads and vegetables. After two weeks, use the Body Monitor Kit to make sure you have determined if you are also suffering from allergies. I also suggest that you take Probiotics and essential fatty acids. (See Chapter 7.) There are tests for *Candida* that can be very valuable. These are provided in Chapter 6.

If your symptoms have not subsided after two weeks, I suggest a stronger anti-*Candida* protocol. If the symptoms start going away, continue this diet for two months. There are many supplements you can take which help rid the body of the excess *Candida*. If you suffer from candidiasis, I recommend that you work with a health professional to determine which supplements might be most appropriate for you.

CANKER SORES AND MOUTH ULCERS

Aphthous Stomatitis, Aphthous Ulceration, Gingivital Ulcers, Oral Ulceration, Recurrent Aphthous Ulcers (RAU), and Ulcerative Sotmatitis

Canker sores are small painful ulcerations that have yellow-gray centers and a red border. They usually occur on mucosa inside the mouth: the inner side of the lips, the tongue, the back and floor of the mouth, and the wall of the cheeks. Canker sores can be single or can occur in clusters, and can be persistent.

The cause of canker sores is uncertain. However, associations with human herpes virus, other viral and/or bacterial infections, local trauma, psychological stress, nutritional deficiencies, food allergies, hormone imbalances, use of medications, and HIV infection have all been suggested as causative factors. Canker sores generally take one to two weeks to heal and may recur monthly or several times per year.[1]

There are many journal articles that show a relationship between canker sores and food allergies.[2] Using the skin prick test (see Chapter 6), which tests for IgE allergic reactions to food, eighteen of the twenty-one patients greatly improved after removal of the allergy-inducing foods.[3] Other research found that gluten-containing foods are associated with recurrent canker sores.[4] The increased antibodies to certain food antigens in some people with recurrent canker sores support the theory of food allergy.[5]

In a study, fifteen patients were tested for gluten, cows' milk protein, three different food colorings, and benzoic acid. Three patients did not finish the study. Six of the patients became symptom-free following removal of cows' milk protein. Eight others showed some improvement.[6] Although no reasons were given as to why people removed themselves from the study, I feel that addictions to wheat and/or milk could have played a role. People are usually not even aware of having an addiction because they eat the food frequently enough so that they do not have to go through withdrawal symptoms. I suspect some patients in the study, having to give up addictive foods, found this difficult and withdrew from the program.

As the research suggests, there could be many causes for canker sores. All of these causes should be looked into. Detoxification is definitely required. Food allergy testing would also be wise for people afflicted with canker sores who have found no other cause.

CYSTIC FIBROSIS (CF)

People with cystic fibrosis (CF) have persistent inflammation that damages the lungs and decreases their ability to fight infection. Many have asthma-like symptoms of shortness of breath and wheezing that accompany the narrowing of airways. Some researchers found respiratory germs to be important causes of inflammation, but they also found that not all respiratory symptoms were due to infection.[1]

Studies show that children with CF were born with normal lungs, but something happened after they were born that caused inflammation and injury. An infection could cause inflammatory mucus that obstructs pancreatic function. Pancreatic enzymes are prevented from reaching the intestines to digest food, causing food allergy. This may explain why individuals with CF often exhibit chronic food allergies. Researchers found that the measurement of antibodies such as IgG was an effective means of diagnosing and treating food allergies occurring with CF. In fact, a diet eliminating foods to which children reacted improved CF symptoms in 90 percent of them.[2] Another study established a direct correlation between raised IgG in the blood and CF. It was concluded that this heightened immune response caused by food allergy could actually worsen the course of the disease.[3]

Still another problem is fungus. Eleven percent of all CF patients have allergic respiratory reactions to the fungus *aspergillus fumigatus.* Pollens and dust mites may also trigger allergic immune response in persons with CF.[4]

Oxidative stress is increased in CF patients, despite normal dietary antioxidant intake. The immune response appears to be a key factor causing oxidative stress. Lipid peroxide is formed in the presence of free radicals. Lipid peroxide levels in CF patients have been carefully studied by researchers, who emphasize that "oxidative stress sustained by CF children must be taken into account so that it does not aggravate the prognosis of the disease."[5] If infection has not been found, it would be wise to test for food allergies using both IgG and IgE methods, chemical sensitivities, free radicals, and fungus. Give the lungs a chance to heal as much as possible as soon as possible.

EPILEPSY

Epilepsy is a brain disorder accompanied by periodic convulsions and loss of consciousness. One of the facts that I have found in more than one study is that when a child has a specific disease, the whole family tends to have more allergies than normal people. The question as to why this happens has to be asked. Many times in these studies, the mother, father, and child or children have allergies. That does not necessarily lead to a conclusion that the child or children inherited allergies. It seems more convincing that a family's eating habits lead to allergies. As we have already discussed, sugar and other junk food can cause allergies that suppress the immune system. Once the immune system is suppressed, a person has a more difficult time fending off both infectious and degenerative diseases.

In one study, epilepsy was the end result, but it might have been any other disease. Dr. Frediani and associates tested the hypothesis that epilepsy is linked to allergy. Their research showed that mothers of an epileptic child had not only higher rates of eczema than the controls, but other family members also had rhinitis and other allergic symptoms. The epileptic children had more asthma, and a significantly higher incidence of allergy to cow's milk in relation to the control group.[1]

There have been other studies that show that there has been improvement or recovery from epileptic seizures as a result of eliminating food allergies. These improvements were most notable in individuals who had additional symptoms such as migraines and digestive problems. Dr. Kinsman used a high fat/low carbohydrate diet with fifty-eight epileptic children who required multiple medications. The research showed that seizure control improved in 67 percent of the children. With this diet, medication could be reduced in 64 percent. Additionally, greater dexterity (36 percent) and improved behavior (23 percent) was noted.[2] When the children followed a low carbohydrate diet, they removed grains, including wheat. I do not think that it was a low carbohydrate diet that improved symptoms; it was removing grains that are highly allergenic to many people. I think that a more thorough testing of food allergies would have resulted in more of the children having fewer seizures.

Oxidative stress also plays a role in seizures. Dr. K. Sudha and his team found that the antioxidant levels in the blood of epileptic patients were low compared to the control group in the study. This study showed that taking antioxidants lowered the number of seizures.[3] Another study showed that taking antioxidants did not help the disease, even though the research showed a low antioxidant level in the bloodstream. The chronic use of antioxidants as antiepileptic agents to help seizures may be detrimental rather than protective.[4] Talk to your health care provider concerning this issue, but it certainly will help to read over all the items that cause oxidative stress and remove as many as possible. For a list of such items, see Chapter 4.

Dr. K. Weber found in epileptic dogs that AGE formation was much faster than in dogs without the disease. Although this was a study with dogs, the theory it produced applies to humans. The pattern of AGE distribution in the brain of a dog is similar to the distribution in a human's brain.[5] It seems logical to remove any item that might cause a seizure, and deal with the stress in your life.

FOOD ADDICTIONS AND EATING DISORDERS
Anorexia, Bulimia, and Compulsive Overeating

An addiction is something that is stronger than a person's willpower to change. In Chapter 3, we demonstrated a causal link between food allergies and addictions. For a time, the body is able to adapt to the allergens produced by addiction, usually because the allergen causes the release of endorphins. Over time, however, the endocrine glands may secrete the wrong amount of hormones, and some minerals may become deficient and others toxic, upsetting body chemistry. Finally, adaptation is no longer possible and degeneration results.

Do you wake up in the morning with headaches and a grouchy demeanor that disappears at breakfast? The people that experience this condition are having withdrawal symptoms, similar to those experienced by heroin addicts, because the endorphins previously present have worn off and need to be replenished by eating a "favorite food." A person with this type of allergic response will crave the foods that he or she is allergic to, because all he or she knows is that the food feels *good* to eat. Yet, the body continues to struggle to adapt to the food, to what it perceives as an "attack," sometimes for years. Eventually, exhaustion will overwhelm the immune system, creating a situation where the allergy surfaces full force, no longer hiding behind symptoms associated with diseases.

After you eat a food or meal, you should feel no better or no worse. If you feel better, you are addicted to the food. If you feel worse, you are allergic to it. Sometimes you can feel better for a few minutes or hours and then feel worse. That is allergy/addiction.

Ideally, after eating you should feel no different, just full. Dr. Hans Seyle observed that people eating something to which they react experience four stages of reaction. First comes an initial acute, alarm reaction, meant to protect the person by creating noticeable symptoms. The mechanism involved in this reaction includes mast cells releasing histamine, which starts the inflammation cycle. Symptoms can strike anywhere in the body, but may include headaches, diarrhea, and drowsiness. If the food is not eaten again, the symptoms go away.

The second stage is known as the addictive stage. In this stage, a person starts craving the food and eats it repeatedly. At this point, he or she is clearly addicted, enjoying the endorphin reaction, but dreading the crash afterwards.

The third stage is called the adaptation stage or the adaptive/addiction stage. If a person consumes the allergen in regular doses to ward off withdrawal, he or she is symptom-free. The homeostasis mechanisms are being challenged, but they are still working. The allergy/addiction becomes firmly rooted over a period of years. At this time, the body says, "Here it comes again. I don't like it but I will adapt." Adapting usually means changes in hormone secretions. For some people, this can mean secreting less than the normal amount of hormone; for others, it can mean secreting too much of a hormone. This is why many people suffer from hormone and endocrine problems. Insulin is one of the hormones that can stop functioning correctly when the body chemistry is continually upset. Is it any wonder why diabetes is the fastest growing disease in America and the rest of the world? Other similar hormonal irregularities and deficiencies may strike the thyroid, sex glands, and adrenal glands. Needless to say, during this stage, the body experiences a state of chronic stress, resulting in a precarious balance.

At any time during the adaptive stage the body may initiate the final stage, known as degeneration. The body can become overloaded with food allergies, environmental allergies, infections, emotional distress, and/or excessive cold, heat, or fatigue, causing the immune system to shut down after years of abuse. The body says, "That's it! I'm depleted and exhausted. Do this stupid job without me!" This four-step cycle of allergy, addiction, adaptation, and degeneration is a root cause of many diseases.[1]

Obesity and Addiction

Often people who eat food to which they are allergic (because of the addictive endorphin rush), eat too much, causing obesity. They think if a little food tastes good, a lot of food tastes better. Addictions to other substances (drugs, alcohol, or tobacco) function the same way. I know of no person addicted to foods to which they are not allergic. I suggest that overweight people remove all forms of sugar, wheat, and dairy products (except butter) from their diet, and watch to see how much weight is lost. Usually the results are surprisingly positive, since these food groups are often the foods to which people are most addicted. Once these three highly addictive food classes are dealt with, other allergies/addictions may surface. Like the Big Bad Three, removing other food allergens from your diet will help you to regain control, or else suffer a relapse of cravings.

Obese people will testify to the overwhelming power of food allergy addiction, as they continue to eat allergenic foods day after day. Such compulsive eaters have no idea that daily food cravings or eating habits result from a physiological and psychological need to stop withdrawal symptoms.[2] A person might have good intentions to stop eating, but when the shakes or headaches start, he or she becomes helpless. As with any kind of pain, a person will do anything to stop the aching, including eating the offending foods again in order to feel better—but in the long run the withdrawal symptoms will return.[3]

Dr. Charles McGee, author of *How to Survive Modern Technology,* expressed his opinion that food and chemical allergies could be a major cause of obesity. He wrote, "There are many people who are addicted to all sorts of foods. People who are addicted to coffee, do not necessarily get fat. If they are addicted to sugar or wheat, they may end up running around with candies or wheat-containing crackers in their pockets to satisfy the craving. What's most important is that it's extremely difficult for these allergic individuals to lose weight unless they ultimately gain control of their food allergies. They must identify the particular allergens, break the craving, and then eliminate the chemical or food."[4]

Scientists at the U.S. Department of Energy's Brookhaven National Laboratory have found that the mere display of food— where food-deprived subjects are allowed to smell and taste their favorite foods without actually eating them—causes a significant elevation in the brain of dopamine, a neurotransmitter associated with feelings of pleasure and reward. "Eating is a highly reinforcing behavior, just like taking illicit drugs," said psychiatrist Nora Volkow, the study's lead investigator. "But this is the first time anyone has shown that the dopamine system can be triggered by food when there is no pleasure associated with it since the subjects don't eat the food. This gives new clues about the mechanisms that lead people to eat other than just for the pleasure of eating, and in this respect may help us understand why some people overeat."[5]

Sugar Addiction

Although the term sugar addiction often appears in magazines and television, until recently scientists had not demonstrated that sugar dependency really exists. But a recent experiment at Princeton University resulted in a clear finding of sugar addiction in rats. Male rats were put on an alternating cycle of twelve hours with food spiked with 25 percent added sugar, and twelve hours of food deprivation, for several days. During the food deprived half-day, the rats showed forms of anxiety such as teeth chattering, forepaw tremor, and head shakes, similar to rats withdrawing from morphine or nicotine.[6] Dr. Philpott speculates that frequent contact with allergenic foods, like sugar, triggers a rise in the brain opioid enkephalin, a narcotic produced by the body that is as addictive as externally supplied narcotics.[7]

I see withdrawal symptoms in many people, and they are never easy to overcome. Whether it is sugar or something else that you are addicted to, do not quit cold turkey; you should employ the gradual step-down system, like with nicotine patches.

If you have cravings you are not alone. Read this testimony.

My son's allergist and his arthritic doctor both said the same thing about craving the foods you are allergic to. My son is highly allergic to milk and has a newly found allergy to wheat also which has a cross-reactivity with cane sugar since it's from the grass grain family. Hmmmm. Any surprise for a kid who craves sweets, cheeses, pizza, etc? Not to me it's not.

This child has too many doctors. Remove junk foods and allergy/

addictive foods and he will not need the doctors. This is just the tip of the iceberg. The child is in for many more symptoms and diseases as an adult, if these problems are not addressed now.

Allergy, Addiction, and Inflammation

It has been stated that food allergy can cause partially digested food in the bloodstream. This becomes an irritant, and inflammation sets in around the partially digested food. Many foods that a person is allergic to are addictive; therefore, inflammation can follow addictions. If the person has been addicted for years, chances are that he or she has also had a low-grade inflammation. Assuming the person is still in the allergy adaptive stage, removing the allergen will clear up the inflammation reasonably quickly. If degeneration has set in, more time will be required to heal.

Eating Disorders

Addictions relate to most eating disorders that involve binge eating (compulsive overeating) because of the dopamine/endorphin reaction. Binge eating and bulimia nervosa (binge eating followed by purging) fit into this category. In both cases, removing reactive foods will aid the psychological treatments usually prescribed. Withdrawal symptoms can be difficult to tolerate, but unless a person is very far along the adaptive stage, the condition lasts only a day or two.

Even the non-addictive allergic reaction has an effect on eating disorders. An allergen can result in a drastic reduction of blood glucose levels, accompanied by weakness, hunger, perspiration, headaches, PMS, exhaustion, and irritability. Allergic hunger does not respond to the brain's satiety mechanisms that tell the body to stop eating when enough regular food has been consumed. This hunger leads to obesity and eating disorders.[8] So, removing substances that cause both the straight allergic reaction and the allergy/addiction reaction make sense when dealing with an eating disorder.

Anorexia nervosa is one of the most common forms of malnutrition observed in Western society in individuals without physical diseases, with an average risk of mortality of 20 percent in a younger population aged between fifteen and twenty-five years. It is characterized by an initial dramatic decrease in food intake that leads to profound depletion in muscle and fat mass. There is a direct correlation between anorexia nervosa and irritable bowel syndrome. (See below for more information on irritable bowel syndrome.) If your gastrointestinal tract hurts when you eat, you are less likely to eat. Since irritable bowel syndrome is directly associated with food allergy, it would be helpful to check a person with anorexia nervosa for food allergies.[9] If the pain goes away, they might be more likely to eat.

Research shows that adolescents with eating disorders are at risk for health problems later in life. Whether these symptoms are psychological like anxiety, depression, and insomnia, or physical like heart problems, infections, and neurological diseases, inflammation is the key factor, as allergy/addiction causes the inflammation.[10] The sooner the eating disorder can be dealt with through psychological and nutritional counseling, the easier it will be on the person and the less possibility there will be of future health problems.

HEADACHES

Cluster, Migraine, Sinus, and Tension Headaches

There is a direct correlation between inflammation and all classes of headaches. The primary types of headaches and their definitions are provided below.

Tension Headache

Inflammation of the blood vessels in the scalp causes tension headaches. Symptoms may include tenderness in the head, muscle aches, and red swollen eyes. This type of headache usually occurs in people over age sixty.

Cluster Headaches

A cluster headache is a rare type of headache that is more common in men. Cluster headaches start suddenly. The pain is usually behind or around one eye and is very severe. The nose and eye on the same side as the pain may become red, swollen, and runny. A cluster headache can last for a few minutes or for several hours, but it usually lasts for thirty to forty-five minutes. These headaches typically occur at the same time each day for several weeks, until the "cluster period" is over. Cluster periods usually last four to eight weeks and may occur every few months. At other times, no cluster headaches will occur.[1]

Sinus Headaches

Sinus headaches are associated with a swelling of the membranes lining the sinuses (spaces adjacent to the nasal passages). Pain occurs in the affected region—the result of air, pus, and mucus being trapped within the obstructed sinuses. Discomfort often occurs under the eye and in the upper teeth (disguised as a headache or toothache). Sinus headaches tend to worsen as you bend forward or lie down. The key to relieving the symptoms is to reduce sinus swelling and inflammation and facilitate mucus drainage from the sinuses.

Migraines

Most of the research on headaches deals with migraines. A migraine is a vascular headache caused by changes in the blood vessels in the head. These headaches arise from several physiological imbalances: inadequate blood supply, low serotonin, platelet disorders (small disks which circulate in blood that help in blood clotting), and nerve disorders. There is a buildup of inflammation-causing substances in the central nervous system.[2]

Headache, Food Allergy, and Chemical Sensitivity

For many people with these symptoms, there is an easy answer. The inflammation-causing substances in the central nervous system are food allergies and chemical sensitivities. Find the foods to which you react, remove them, and the headaches go away. Reintroduce the foods and the headaches return. For some it could be as easy as eliminating one food, for others it may be a variety of foods. Although much of the research correlates food and chemical allergies with migraine headaches, this information can apply to any headache.

Researchers who conducted a double-blind, placebo-controlled study found that eighty-two of eighty-eight migraine headache sufferers experienced noticeable relief of symptoms with the identification and elimination of both food allergens and chemical additives from their diet. Usually, multiple foods were involved. Most of the responses were delayed in onset, ranging from one hour to three days. The symptoms took anywhere from one to twenty-one days to improve. Most were not identified or suspected by the patients or their relatives. Not only did migraines disappear, so did associated symptoms, such as diarrhea, cramping, flatulence, behavioral disorders, epilepsy, limb aches and pains, eczema, asthma, and mouth ulcers. The researchers found that allergy correlated with many different symptoms and diseases. The authors conclude that IgE testing is valuable but may not reveal all allergenic foods.[3] Adding IgG testing to the arsenal would have found more allergy foods. (See Chapter 6.)

Pediatric specialists from the Department of Neurology at the Hospital for Sick Children in London have performed a number of studies on migraines in children over the years. In one study, they found that 93 percent of children improved with a diet that avoided offending foods. Later they examined forty-five epileptic children with migraines and/or hyperactive behavior. Headaches, seizures, and hyperactive behavior were eradicated in twenty-five children and reduced in eleven others after eliminating reactive foods.[4] As this research shows, resolving the food allergy relieved many other symptoms in these children besides headaches. Rarely do you see articles in magazines and newspapers concerning the relationship between migraines and food allergies. I think this is a large piece of the puzzle that needs addressing.

Dr. Ellen Grant found that chemicals in the home environment can also cause headache symptoms. When a person is very sensitive, it is important to remove as many of the foods and chemicals as possible to give a person's immune system a chance to heal. Grant found that both IgE (immediate) and IgG (delayed) reactions were involved in allergic reactions. She also noted that other provocative allergens were cigarettes and birth control pills. She believes that there is strong evidence for the allergic causation of high blood pressure, arthritis, asthma, and diabetes.[5] See these sections in this book for more information on this theory.

Some headaches are provoked by food additives or naturally-occurring food chemicals, such as monosodium glutamate (often added to Asian food and packaged foods), tyramine (found in many cheeses), phenylethylamine (found in chocolate), or alcohol. The artificial sweetener aspartame has also been reported to trigger migraines in some people. The chemicals that free radicals produce can go to the brain causing migraines and other headaches.[6]

Psychological Stress

The "fight or flight" reaction can also lead to headaches. This reaction can be triggered by actual or merely perceived challenges, dangers, or invasions. The brain releases adrenaline during the fight or flight response. The adrenaline produces energy in the muscles and nerves that trigger other chemicals that lead to inflammation and pain. This is the key to understanding how stress, which is strictly mental, can lead to physical manifestations as inflammation and pain. How you view a situation is more important than the situation itself.[7] Complications arise when a stressful event is perceived as a distressful situation. Just by thinking something stressful, inflammation and pain can set in, not only in the head, but in other parts of the body, as well.

Where one feels the pain varies from individual to individual based on his or her genetic blueprint. If the pain occurs in the head, it can develop in the temples, neck, forehead, or all over. The muscles in the shoulders and neck can hurt in tension headaches. But tension that causes inflammation can develop anywhere throughout the body, causing pain. If you have reoccurring headaches of any sort, it would be wise to learn the skills of relaxation and stress management.[8] All people with headaches need to address what they eat, as well as what they feel, think, say, and do. What you eat can affect how your head feels and what you think and feel can affect your whole body.

HEARTBURN

Acid Reflux Disease, Eosinophilic Esophagitis, Esophagitis, and Gastroesophageal Reflux Disease (GERD)

The terms above all refer to the presence of inflammation somewhere in the gastrointestinal tract, commonly known as heartburn. Heartburn is caused when stomach acid flows upward (reflux) from the stomach into the esophagus, the tube that carries food from the throat to the stomach. This occurs when the lower esophageal sphincter, the ring of muscles at the lower end of the esophagus, fails to keep the esophagus properly closed. When it is functioning properly, this sphincter relaxes to allow food to pass through to the stomach, but otherwise remains constricted. When stomach acid comes in contact with the walls of the esophagus, an uncomfortable pain or burning sensation behind the sternum can result, sometimes radiating toward the mouth, neck, or throat. As the backup of acid flows from the stomach into the esophagus, irritation and inflammation occur. Dr. Marc Rothenberg, of the Children's Hospital Medical Center in Cincinnati, Ohio, found that when people are treated for asthma, the condition of their esophagus improves. He believes that there is a connection between the development of food and environmental allergies, and esophagitis.[1]

The best way of curbing heartburn pain is not using antacids, but changing your diet. I suggest you follow my Food Plan III (see Chapter 7), and test yourself to make sure you have found all of your allergies. You can do this simply and effectively, using my Body Monitor Kit (see Chapter 6).

Each person is different, and so is each allergy. Dr. Rothenberg found that allergies related to esophagitis were not classical allergies. Rather, they were chronic in nature and most likely IgG-mediated, not IgE-mediated, thus usually not detected by doctors using conventional allergy tests.

There are some things you can do to relieve the symptoms of heartburn. Instead of eating three large meals daily, eat smaller, more frequent meals every two to three hours, following Food Plan III. Eat your food slowly and chew it well. Get in the habit of putting down your fork after every bite and chewing at least ten times. Both of these suggestion will help, but if you do not remove the offending food or foods causing the problem, the problem will not go away.

HEART DISEASE

Angina, Arteriosclerosis, Atherosclerosis, Cardiomyopathy, Coronary Artery Disease, Coronary Heart Disease, Endocarditis, Ischemic Heart Disease, Myocardial Infarction, Myocarditis, Pericarditis, and Stroke

The Dictionary of Science defines heart disease as any ailment of the heart or coronary arterial system. The mainstream medical community has begun publishing articles showing that inflammation, rather than cholesterol, is the key indicator of risk of heart disease. My studies on the subject led me to the conclusion that the researchers were covering old ground.

In the late nineteenth century, German physiologist Rudolph Virchow (1821–1902) proposed that heart disease was caused by inflammation of the heart and the arterial plumbing that serves the heart.

He came to this conclusion by observing that the hearts of people who had died of heart disease looked like bruised and infected flesh.[1] Then the idea was dropped for some time.

Briefly revived in the twentieth century, the inflammation link turned out to be a flash in the pan as doctors focused instead on low-fat diets and cholesterol-reducing drugs. This line of experimentation worked to some degree, but half of all heart attacks and strokes occur in people with normal cholesterol. By the 1980s, researchers re-examined inflammation as a cause. Dr. Peter Libby took arterial cells from rabbits and irritated them with a bacterial toxin causing a release of inflammatory cytokines. Testing human tissues with similar toxins found a similar cytokine release.[2]

Despite lifestyle changes and effective cholesterol drugs, heart disease remains a major killer in the developed world, but not in developing nations. Cholesterol screening fails to identify 50 percent of those people with acute conditions. In the case of atherosclerosis, new research demonstrates that the disease is more than a problem of lipid deposits in the cardio-pulmonary (heart and lung) system; it is also an inflammatory process.

Gradually, researchers have assembled a new model for heart attacks and strokes that suggests that inflammatory immune-system cells burrow into an arterial wall and consume fat droplets. These cells form a plaque that is weakened by inflammation. Then the fibrous cap ruptures, spilling everything into the bloodstream, including cytokines that encourage blood clotting. The artery fills up with rapidly coagulating blood cells that may block the vessel, causing heart attacks and strokes. Thus, a stable cholesterol plaque is changed to an unstable lesion (injury). "This is an idea that has emerged in a popular way in only the last few years," Libby said. "The blood vessel is a living breathing organ, and the plaque is not just a graveyard for cholesterol debris; it's teeming with cells."[3]

A primary goal of heart attack prevention, according to Libby and others, is a reduction of inflammation, one indicator of which is C-reactive protein (CRP). Researchers have not fully explained the mechanism linking CRP to heart disease, but there is a connection. CRP has become the accepted inflammation marker for heart disease as well as other diseases. As a health precaution, consider having your physician test your CRP levels. (See Chapter 6.)

Generalized edema often goes ignored in many cases while

blood vessel walls develop leaks as the disease progresses. A low-grade chronic swelling and inflammation may loosen fatty plaque, which may lodge in arteries and obstruct blood flow.[4] According to Dr. Paul Ridker, high levels of CRP are a good predictor of heart disease; it is even better than low-density lipoprotein (LDL) cholesterol.

Obesity

Obesity plays a major role in the CRP model of heart disease. The best methods of losing weight—changing diets and exercising—are also the best ways to lower CRP. Also give up smoking. Researchers found that the risks of heart disease for overweight people to be 34 percent greater than non-overweight individuals. More frightening, the risks for obese people were 104 percent greater.[5]

Angina

Unstable angina, chest pain due to heart disease and blocked arteries, may result from inflammation caused by an immune response. A research team lead by Dr. G. Caliguri found higher levels of inflammatory markers during acute illness in patients with unstable angina than those with stable angina (chest pains due to exercise). The researchers speculated that the problem may be triggered by an antigen, but could not identify the specific one. An unknown antigen suggests food allergies, AGEs, and free radicals could be a cause of the condition. The stronger the inflammation and immune response, the more violent symptoms the person will feel.[6]

Sugar and the Gylcemic Load

Dr. John Yudkin, an English medical doctor, proposes that sugar is a cause of heart disease.[7] He found that healthy middle-aged women of normal weight who consumed large quantities of sugar had high CRP levels. The inflammatory marker CRP is elevated in heart patients; therefore, sugar increases the risk of heart disease.[8]

Infections

Many studies suggest that common viral and bacterial infections raise the risk of heart disease. Various culprits include herpes simplex one (cold sores), cytomeglovirus (a virus with no known symptoms), gum disease (bacteria), *H. Pylori* (ulcers),[9] and *Chlamydia Pneumoniae* (bronchitis and pneumonia), which have all been found in arterial plaques.[10] It is not yet clear that any of these infections directly irritate artery walls, so researchers call it an unfinished theory. A German study headed by Dr. C. Espinola-Klein showed a direct relationship between infections and atherosclerosis. Moreover, the risk of death increased by the number of infectious pathogens present, especially in patients with advanced atherosclerosis.[11]

Dr. A. F. Stone suggests that infection sets off the body's inflammatory responses, similar to smoking, obesity, and arthritis. Dr. David Siskovich regards such findings as preliminary, but generally agrees that infections play a role in heart disease.[12] There are no known bacterial relationships to atherosclerosis, which explains the general futility of antibiotics for reducing risks. However, anti-inflammatory drugs used for arthritis and similar conditions have been used successfully.[13] Again, it seems more logical to find out what is causing the inflammation so it can be removed from the body, rather than to simply take a drug.

High Blood Pressure (Hypertension)

High blood pressure (hypertension) afflicts about 50 million Americans, many of whom are not aware that they suffer from it, or of the toll it can take on health. High blood pressure elevates cytokine production and amplifies the inflammatory response, according to Dr. Claudia U. Chae. Again, the mechanism is unclear, but there is no question that hypertension and heart disease are directly related. The risks apply even to those with "high normal" blood pressure.[14]

Sometimes the truth sneaks in the back door. Dr. Ellen Grant studied migraines and food allergy, discovering that most of her subjects' symptoms cleared up after removing allergens. Twenty-five percent of her subjects also had high blood pressure, which also improved by removing allergens.[15] High blood pressure is just one way an allergic stress shows up in your body.

High blood pressure has long been linked to obesity and smoking, both of which, in turn, are linked to inflammation. New research shows that there is compelling evidence that inflammation is also a likely contributing factor to high blood pressure, even in the absence of obesity and smoking. In one study, researchers measured CRP in over 20,000 healthy women. They monitored the women, who were all aged 45 and over, for nearly eight years to see who would develop high blood pressure of at least 140/90, the established cutoff for hypertension. During that period, 5,365 women became hypertensive.

Women who came into the study with high levels of CRP but no apparent disease, had a 52 percent greater risk of developing high blood pressure. This research was part of the ongoing Woman's Health Study headed by Howard D. Sesso, an epidemiologist at Brigham and Women's Hospital in Boston. Some studies suggest that elevated CRP indicates that blood vessels are already damaged.[16] In addition, CRP levels are associated with the future development of hypertension, which also indicates that hypertension is in part an inflammatory disorder.

Food Allergy

Inflamed veins, usually in the legs due to a thrombus (blood clot) earned the name thrombophlebitis (blood clots in inflammation), and may be caused by chemicals, bacteria, or an unknown cause. Dr. William Rea found that this unknown agent could be food allergy. He studied ten patients experiencing calf pain and tenderness using extensive environmental control methods. All patients became symptom-free of their phlebitis without medication, but eight had symptoms return after allergens were reintroduced. Both inhaled chemicals and allergic foods caused symptoms.[17]

Another study included twelve patients with irregular heart beat and/or chest pain. The symptoms cleared in ten patients without medication when chemicals and foods to which they reacted were removed. When the patients were reintroduced to the allergic substances, the symptoms returned. Inflammation played a role because both complement and lymphocytes were activated.[18]

AGEs

AGEs also seem to play a role in heart disease. In one study, blood concentrations of AGEs were significantly higher in non-diabetic subjects with coronary artery disease than in control subjects. The diet was not discussed in this study, but the authors said that the greater the AGEs concentrations, the greater the vascular damage.[19] In the next study we can see that restricting the amount of AGEs in the diet restricts arterial damage, as well.

Dr. Helen Vlassara led a team that studied the effects of two diets on inflammatory markers on twenty-four patients with diabetes. One diet included a diet high in AGEs and the other had low amounts. Diets high in AGEs create a constant state of low-grade inflammation, damaging small to mid-sized arteries and leading to heart disease. When AGEs in the diet were restricted, there was less arterial damage.[20] If you suffer from heart disease, it would be wise to again read through the section on AGEs in Chapter 4 to find out what foods to eliminate that cause AGEs. I will give you a clue, sugar is the most important food to eliminate. Read Food Plan III in Chapter 7 to find out what foods you can safely consume.

Free Radicals and Oxidative Stress

Oxidative stress can manifest in heart disease when blood vessels make too many free radicals. Oxidation depletes important nutrients, leading to plaque formation. Additionally, strong evidence exists showing that free radicals oxidize LDL (low density lipoproteins), which are consumed by white blood cells to form plaque on the cardiovascular wall. Blood vessels harden and narrow, impairing blood flow and starving the heart of oxygen and nutrients.[21]

Unknown Origin

Researchers do not yet agree on the causes, so phrases like "unknown origin" and "unfinished theory" litter their research publications, suggesting a missing link. Dr. R. P. Tracy says that heart inflammation is similar to arthritis,[22] a condition with a well-documented relationship to food allergy.[23] Eliminating food allergies is a good first step to preventing or healing heart disease, but all the factors in this section have to be considered, including stress from long hours of work, too little sleep,[24] lack of exercise, anger, and depression.

INFLAMMATORY BOWEL DISEASE (IBD)

Celiac Disease, Crohn's Disease, Functional Colitis, Functional Gastrointestinal Disorders or Bowel Disorders, Gastroenteritis, Irritable Bowel Syndrome (IBS), Nervous Indigestion, Spastic Colon, and Ulcerative Colitis

Irritable bowel syndrome (IBS) is a multi-factorial gastrointestinal condition affecting 8–22 percent of the population, with a higher prevalence in women. It is characterized by abdominal pain, excessive gas, alternating diarrhea and constipation, and abdominal bloating for which there is no evidence of detectable organic disease.[1] Many people suffer through frequent relapses. Names of IBS vary depending on where the inflammation strikes and the severity of the condition, but for our purposes they are all similar diseases. The causes are thought to be multifactorial, involving diet, infection, antibiotics, and psychological stress.

Food Allergies

Many researchers have found that food allergies can cause inflammatory bowel disease. Using skin test, IgE test, and IgG test on IBD sufferers, researchers found that the IgG test showed the most allergies that related to the IBD symptoms, although this test is done the least when testing for food allergies.[2] Sugar, wheat, dairy, corn, fish, peanuts, and eggs were common inducers of IBS.[3] The treatment for IBS is usually aimed at controlling symptoms. However, evaluation of food allergy may provide a useful adjunct in those with severe symptoms or a clear history of adverse food reaction.[4]

Sugar

Are we clear on my position that sugar wrecks mineral balance, leading to all sorts of diseases? In people with IBD, sugar can more than upset body chemistry. Dr. R. Goldstein and associates found that lactose, fructose, and sorbitol impair intestinal absorption of nutrients (malabsorption). Removing all sugars, including the previous list and glucose, sucrose, honey, maple syrup, corn syrup, and fructose, improved symptoms.[5]

Stress

As repeatedly demonstrated throughout this book, stress or, rather, the perception of stress, plays a role in all diseases. This is certainly true for IBD. Stress management therapy can help reduce complaints and symptoms.[6]

Antibiotics

Antibiotic usage is arduous for patients with IBD, as people taking those drugs are three times as likely to report bowel symptoms compared to normal, even four months after terminating the drug.[7] The more you keep your body in homeostasis, the less likely you will have to take antibiotics.

MMR and Measles Virus

Recent research postulates a link between measles virus, MMR (measles, mumps, and rubella vaccine), and inflammatory bowel disease in adults.[8] If a person has IBD and has had the measles or MMR, it is important to keep the body in homeostasis as much as possible. The immune system is already compromised as it is.

Some research shows an overload of various factors can cause symptoms.[9] A little stress, a little sugar, a few rounds of antibiotics, and the body says "Adios Amigo." The immune system can no longer deal with the overload and inflammation and eventually disease sets in.

Probiotics

Our body has natural healthy bacteria that are essential for intestinal health and homeostasis. When the intestinal wall becomes inflamed, the good bacteria are depleted, and need to be replaced. Research has shown that taking probiotics will help maintain the balance of the intestinal microflora (good bacteria and fungi) and alleviate many of the symptoms of IBD.[10] (See Chapter 7.) Moreover, studies have suggested that probiotics are as effective as anti-spasmodic drugs in the alleviation of IBD.[11]

Celiac Disease (Coeliac Disease, Celiac Sprue, and Gluten Intolerance)

Recent research has shown that there is also a relationship between celiac disease and IBD.[12] Celiac disease is a disorder that causes bowel irritation, bloating, cramps, inflammation, diarrhea, malnutrition, depression, respiratory infections, and weight loss. In children, it may also delay or inhibit puberty and stunt growth. The main reason is a sensitivity to gluten, found in wheat, rye, oats, barley, kamut, and spelt. Kamut and spelt (products found in health food stores) are variants of wheat. Unfortunately gluten can be used as a filler found in dairy products, chocolate, canned foods, and processed foods. Read your labels.

Other conditions can also develop, including neurological problems and/or dermatitis herpetiformis (blister-like lesions on the elbows, buttocks, and knees). This disease doubles patients' risk of death for all diseases. Those patients who are not diagnosed until they have had the disease for a period of time or do not adhere to a strict diet free of gluten, are at most risk for many problems down the road.

Celiac disease has brought attention to the role that food can play in the disease process. Dr. Giovanni Corrao and a research team studied the death rate of 1,072 adults with celiac disease from 1962 to1994. The results were astounding, finding that the mortality rate was twice that of the control group who did not have celiac disease. The causes of death include: cancer, circulatory, respiratory, and digestive diseases. Delayed diagnosis, because of symptomless early forms of the disease, poor adherence to a gluten-free diet, and severe symptoms all relate to the high death rate.[13] Limited thinking sometimes makes things worse. Celiac disease is not just about gluten intolerance, but may also incorporate other allergies the patient may have. Therefore, a total food allergy panel should be used when testing for celiac disease.

Diseases Concurrent with Celiac Disease

Celiac disease has been diagnosed in patients with other diseases. Still other times low-grade inflammation continues in the intestinal tract and throughout the body for many years, with gluten intolerance undiagnosed. The following are some of the diseases that are connected to gluten intolerance.

1. People with celiac disease often develop cancers of the intestines. The leading cause of death from cancer is non-Hodgkin's lymphoma.[14]

2. Asthma, hay fever, and eczema were significantly more common in patients with adult celiac disease than in normal controls.[15]

3. Type I Diabetes, childhood diabetes, is associated with gluten intolerance.[16]

4. Arthritis is linked to people with celiac disease.[17]

5. Systemic lupus erythematous (lupus) is associated with a wheat intolerance.[18]

6. Autistic disorders and attention deficit disorders are now being linked with gluten intolerance.

7. Fibromyalgia, chronic fatigue syndrome, and gulf war syndrome all have symptoms that are the same as celiac disease.[19]

8. Depression and panic disorder are both connected to gluten sensivity. [20]

9. Headaches can be from gluten intolerance. Inflammation in the central nervous system causes the headaches.[21]

10. Psoriasis conditions improve when people with this condition go on a gluten-free diet.[22]

11. Many people with Hashimoto's thyroiditis, an autoimmune thyroid disease, were found to have a wheat intolerance.[23]

Celiac disease is thought to be genetic. However, this idea does not corroborate with the fact that in China and Japan, where rice is the main staple, celiac disease is rare.[24] There are some scientists that say wheat should not be eaten by anyone. I'm not sure if it is the properties in wheat that can be debilitating for many, many people, or that many have abused wheat by eating it with sugar (cookies, cake, donuts, Danish, pie, and muffins). The *Archives of Internal Medicine* published an article stating that celiac disease occurs frequently not only in patients with gastrointestinal symptoms, but also in first- and second-degree relatives and patients with numerous common disorders even in the absence of gastrointestinal symptoms.[25] I do know that many people could have symptoms eliminated by not eating wheat. If you have unresolved symptoms you might remove all gluten from your diet for a week and see what happens. But, as I have stated, you are wasting your time if you do not remove sugar also.

KIDNEY DISEASE

Chronic Renal Failure, Glomerular Nephritis, and Idiopathic Nephrotic Syndrome

Kidney disease is marked by inflammation, vomiting, infections, weight gain despite normal calorie intake, eyelid edema, and protein in the urine.[1] Blood in the urine causing anemia is a symptom of acute kidney disease. Doctors call it kidney disease but the symptoms are certainly systemic.

Kidney disease is thought to be the result of antibody-antigen reactions that localize in the kidneys because of their filtering function. The antibody-antigen reaction can be a reaction to germs, chemicals, and/or food. Many medical journal articles show food allergies to be a causative factor.[2] Researchers Dr. A. Kay and Dr. A. Ferguson conclude from investigation that the immune response to a food antigen, causing inflammation, can produce kidney damage. These researchers state: "This intolerance to food antigens may cause partially digested food particles to enter the bloodstream which stimulate an abnormal inflammatory reaction in any target organ, including the kidneys."[3]

In one study, after eliminating cow's milk, symptoms in four out of six children went away. When milk was reintroduced acute symptoms returned.[4] I feel that if the other two children, who did not respond, had been tested for other food allergies, and if those allergy-inducing foods were eliminated, all the children would have returned to normal. In another report, a six-year-old girl with dermatitis, celiac disease, and kidney disease showed a complete resolution of all three conditions after removing gluten from her diet.[5]

There is enough evidence in all this research to show that food allergy plays a significant role in kidney disease. Although wheat and dairy can play a considerable part in the disease process, any other food can also be a problem. Food allergy should be first on a list of possible causes when the cause of kidney disease is unknown.

Dr. N. Selvaraj and associates showed that there was increased oxidative stress which promoted AGEs in patients with chronic kidney failure who were not diabetic nor on dialysis.[6] If you have kidney disease, find a doctor who will deal with food allergy, free radicals, and AGEs, not by giving medicine, but by eliminating everything that could be causing the problem. There are many things that can be done to stop the cause of the disease. In the meantime go on Food Plan III and a vegetarian diet until you are in the hands of a doctor who understands the role that food plays in kidney disease.

OBESITY

The section will be of great interest to over 62 percent of the people reading this book, as they are affected by this subject: overweight and obesity. Americans grow fatter with each passing year, accumulating pounds at even younger ages. The statistics alone could scare ten pounds off of you.

1. Twenty-seven percent of U.S. adults today are obese by the time they reach their mid-30s, about twice the rate as that of the early 1960s.

2. Sixty-one percent of U.S. adults are either overweight or obese. Obesity is defined as a body mass index (BMI) of at least 30. (See below.)

3. Women and ethnic minorities are at increased risk of obesity.

4. People born in 1964 are becoming obese 26 to 28 percent faster than those born in 1957.

5. The International Obesity Task Force estimates 300 million people worldwide are obese.

6. In the United States, obesity is implicated in the deaths of 300,000 people annually from heart disease, stroke, diabetes, cataracts,[1] osteoarthritis,[2] periodontal disease,[3] and cancer.[4]

The first five findings are based on information from more than 9,000 people living in the United States, who reported their height and weight to researchers twelve times over a seventeen-year period. Because people tend to underestimate their weight, the results of the study may be conservative, the researchers note.

Another illness linked to obesity is Parkinson's disease (PD). Excessive weight during middle age may predict development of PD later in life. Almost 8,000 men in Hawaii, aged 45 to 68 and without PD, were evaluated for body mass index and skin fold thickness at the back of the arm and under the shoulder blade. These are all indicators of body fat. Over a thirty-year period, PD developed in 137 men. The risk of PD was three times greater in the men with the highest body fat, and this was independent of physical activity or fat and calorie intake.[5]

Body Mass Index (BMI)

BMI measures a person's weight in relation to his or her height, more accurately predicting risks of weight-related medical complications and a better indicator than weight alone. The higher your BMI, the higher your inflammation level as measured by the blood test for C-reactive protein (CRP).[6] Multiply body weight in pounds by 705. Divide the resulting number by height in inches. Then divide a second time by height in inches. Normal BMI is 20–25. People with a BMI of 25 to 30 are overweight, and 30 or over should be considered obese. You can read more about the BMI on the web at www.halls.md/body-mass-index/bmirefs.htm.

Obesity and Inflammation

Obesity and inflammation relate to each other because fat cells release cytokines that produce inflammation. A group of obese women significantly lowered their cytokine levels by losing 10 percent of their body fat. Obese adults may suffer from potentially dangerous, chronic low-grade inflammation more than average-weight people, according to a large-scale retrospective study of Americans.[7]

Another recent controlled study of 159 men (aged 22 to 63) also found a significant relationship between CRP levels and body fat, including body mass index, waist measurement, and visceral adipose fat (fat detected by a type of body scan called tomography).[8] *Pediatrics* (a medical journal) showed obese children, aged 8 to 16, have higher concentrations of CRP, suggesting a state of low-grade inflammation.[9] The research shows that the more weight women, men, and children have over the normal weight, the more health problems they can have.

According to studies, including one led by Dr. I. Lemieux in the U.S. and another conducted in Britain, fat tissue that develops in the abdomen may be the greatest inflammatory worry. Lemieux feels that as fat increases around the mid-section, cytokines increase, become more active, and CRP levels creep upward.[10] Research in Britain also correlated higher blood levels of CRP with central obesity. Signs of insulin resistance also showed up in the study. High levels of CRP could account for as much as 14 percent of an increased risk for coronary disease, the researchers said.[11] If your weight gain typically hits you around your abdomen and chest, then lower your weight into the normal range as soon as possible.

Research shows that obese people have higher insulin, glucose, and estrogen levels, all of which are also tickets to inflammation. The National Cancer Institute evaluated research from many sources and made statements showing breast, endometrial, colon, kidney, gas-trointestinal, pancreatic, gallbladder, prostate, and ovarian cancer are more prevalent in obese people.[12] Unfortunately, even people who are not obviously overweight may still have disproportionately too much fat. Keep your waist size below 40 inches for men and 32 inches for women, or increased cytokine secretion and inflammation may result even with a normal BMI.[13]

Food Allergies and Obesity

Food allergies hinder weight loss efforts because people crave the very foods to which they react. Our bodies release endorphins ("feel good" chemicals) when partially digested food gets into the bloodstream and causes inflammation. Needing that high from endorphins more and more, people eat more of the allergen, past the level where the body can metabolize it, causing weight gain. Removing those fast foods and foods to which you are specifically allergic/addicted will go a long way towards improving your health. To learn how to do so, see Food Plan III on page 133.

PARKINSON'S DISEASE (PD)

Parkinson's disease is characterized by inflammation involving the microgial cells, which normally fight off infections, but have recently been found to be associated with the death of essential dopamine-producing cells in the brain. If it is possible to reduce the inflammation, it will enable the damaged cells to start to produce dopamine. The late onset and slow-progressing nature of PD has prompted the consideration of different lifestyle factors that cause the inflammation. One of these is multiple chemical sensitivity (MCS), a condition where previous exposure to hydrophobic organic solvents or pesticides appears to render people hypersensitive to a wide range of chemicals. Other exposures can be pharmaceutical drugs and industrial solvents. Persons who use pesticides in their homes are twice as likely to develop PD as people who are not exposed to pesticides.[1] A combination of different pesticides is even more likely to create greater toxicity issues than an individual chemical. Early-life occurrence of inflammation in the brain, as a consequence of either brain injury or exposure to infectious agents, might also be a factor in the disease.[2]

Oxidation and free radicals cause damage to lipids, proteins, and DNA in PD.[3] Different metals can also cause chemical changes in the brain that lead to the death of dopamine-producing cells and inflammation. The passage of toxic chemicals into the brain is greatly facilitated by aluminum. The brain is normally protected from undesirable chemicals that are in the bloodstream by a filter barrier (the blood-brain barrier).[4]

High levels of aluminum have been shown to allow toxic chemicals to cross the blood-brain barrier that would otherwise have been filtered out.[5] Deterioration of the brain is also caused by the accumulation of heavy metals, such as cadmium, lead, and mercury.[6] Additionally, the presence of multiple toxic metals in the brain greatly increases the potential for harmful effects.

Iron overload can intensify Parkinson's disease. Not only do Parkinson's patients have low levels of natural antioxidants, such as glutathione and superoxide dismutase (SOD), but they may also have high levels of iron in the brain.[7] Research shows that taking supplements of antioxidants does not help with PD. Look to your diet.

Elevated copper is often associated with PD, as well. In one study, copper levels were significantly higher in the cerebrospinal fluid of patients with PD than in the control group.[8] Although the specific reason for elevated copper levels was not known, copper is generally high when there is chronic inflammation, such as that caused by autoimmune or undetected allergy reactions.

Drugs, such as aspirin, as well as allergic inflammation of the intestinal wall, allow partly digested food fragments, as well as bacterial endotoxins to be absorbed.[9] The partially digested food and bacterial endotoxins eventually reach the brain, where they act as neurotoxins. If the body is sufficiently sensitive (particularly as it is in young children), neurotoxins tend to produce acute psychotic symptoms. In persons of advancing age, neurotoxins more commonly cause chronic nerve and brain degeneration. Another common source of endotoxins is from a root canal procedure, from otherwise diseased teeth, or from jawbone cavitations resulting from the extraction of infected teeth.[10]

Excitotoxins are taste or flavor enhancers that release glutamate and other brain-active amino acids, such as aspartate and cysteine. The best known example of an excitotoxin is monosodium glutamate (MSG). High blood levels of MSG can cross the normally protective blood-brain barrier. Glutamate is a neurotransmitter that is present in the extracellular fluid in very low concentrations. If glutamine levels are inappropriately raised, neurons fire abnormally and at higher levels, and brain cells begin to die.[11]

Most processed foods contain excitotoxins, especially any type of commercial taste or flavor enhancer, such as hydrolyzed vegetable protein, soy protein extract, and yeast extract. These are found in beef stock, commercial soups, sauces, gravies, caseinate, and aspartame. These excitotoxins may simply be labeled as "natural" flavorings. Red meat, processed meat, cheeses, and tomato puree have higher levels of glutamate, as well. All processed foods should be avoided by persons with PD.[12] Undetected food allergies and chemical sensitivities contribute to the development of many degenerative diseases. Additionally, we know that the intestinal tract becomes increasingly inefficient with advancing age and degenerative diseases, as well as from allergic inflammation, aspirin use, and absorption of endotoxins and partially digested food as noted earlier.

It has been known for many years that immune system alterations occur in PD. Changes occur in lymphocyte populations in cerebrospinal fluid and in blood and T-cell activation. There is also an increase in cytokines. PD patients exhibit a lower frequency of infections and cancer, suggesting that immune system stimulation may occur.[13] Food allergies and chemical sensitivities may manifest as higher L-dopamine requirements, gradual worsening symptoms, or increasing dysfunctional periods. Detrimental effects are also seen from a high intake of sugar and fat. A diet that is high in sugar increases the risk of developing PD threefold.[14] A diet that includes high levels of animal fat is also associated with a fivefold increase.[15]

Although there could be many causes of PD, exposure to chemicals and allergic foods, combined with a weakness of the detoxifying ability of the liver and a deficiency of antioxidant protection of the brain are usually involved. This results in deterioration of energy metabolism in the brain and makes the dopamine system susceptible to chemical and emotional stress. Other factors include an accident involving the back of the head or the spine (usually involving an injury) or displacement of the atlas or top, vertebra, with accompanying blocking of the flow of cerebrospinal fluid or acupuncture energies.

To reverse these conditions, detoxify the body by:

• Minimizing further chemical damage.

- Improving brain metabolism by removing allergic food and eating only whole foods. There are specific nutrients that work for certain people. It would be wise to explore these supplements.

- Correcting any spinal damage.

- Restoring energy flows in the acupuncture meridians to and from the brain.

PERIODONTAL DISEASE
Gingivitis, Gum Disease, Periodontitis, and Pyorrhea

Periodontal disease affects between 10 and 15 percent of people worldwide. In the United States, 15 percent of adults aged 21 to 50 and 30 percent of people over the age of 50 suffer from severe periodontal disease. Over time, complications from periodontal disease may force a person to lose his or her teeth.[1] The inflammation associated with periodontal disease develops as a result of bacterial infection from a build-up of the sticky, colorless bacterial plaque that continually forms on the surface of the teeth, and especially in the crevices between them. The inflammation that results from such infection is characterized by pain, loose teeth, bleeding, and swelling of the gums. This inflammation also destroys the attachment fibers and supporting bone that hold the teeth in the mouth. Periodontal disease can be treated non-surgically or, in severe cases, with surgery.

Over the years studies have suggested an association between human periodontal disease and certain systemic disorders, such as diabetes mellitus, pneumonia, heart disease, and stroke, all of which are related to systemic inflammation. Periodontal disease is also associated with pre-term birth (see page 105). New data suggest that this association is not indicated by traditional clinical signs of periodontal disease, but rather by inflammatory white blood cells throughout the body that come with periodontal disease.[2]

A study from the University of Birmingham in England examined twenty subjects for the levels of glutathione (an antioxidant): ten of the subjects had healthy gums and ten had advanced gum disease. Samples of a fluid that is routinely released from the crevice within the gums were studied. All the subjects with periodontal disease had substantially lower levels of glutathione in the fluid. When blood serum levels were tested for glutathione, the same disparity was recorded for the two groups. The food sources that have glutathione precursors are meats, fresh fruits, and fresh vegetables. Unfortunately, oral supplements will not help because the molecules are too big to pass through the intestinal walls to the bloodstream.[3] Since this research shows that an antioxidant is deficient in those with periodontal diseases, it would be wise to make sure that the free radicals are controlled. (See Chapter 4 and Chapter 7.) Also make sure you eat meats, fresh fruits, and fresh vegetables.

Gentle mastication (chewing) is able to induce the release of bacterial endotoxins from the mouth into the bloodstream, especially when patients have severe periodontal disease. The periodontium (fibrous connective tissue surrounding the root of a tooth that separates it from, and attaches it to, the alveolar bone) can become diseased. The periodontium can be a major and underestimated source of chronic, or even permanent, release of bacterial pro-inflammatory components into the bloodstream. The whole body can become involved. The problem can become systemic so get it under control.

The impact of stress on the immune system has been well-established. Emotional stress represents a risk indicator for periodontal disease and should be addressed before and during dental treatment.[4] Food allergy has also been implicated in gingivitis, the beginning stages of periodontal disease. In one study, removing reactive foods made treatment more effective.[5] It seems that bacteria must have help to do harm; stress, smoking, chewing gum, and food allergies can create the stage for bacterial infection. Certainly seeing a dentist at least twice a year, brushing your teeth twice a day and flossing are important, but dealing with the other reasons why you have symptoms or illnesses will be helpful for removing periodontal disease. Removing periodontal disease can help with other diseases. It is a holistic approach.

Chewing Gum

While we are on the subject of mouth disease that may result in surgery, chewing gum and tobacco seem logical subjects. Investigators studied the linkage between endotoxins (those chemicals that initiate inflammation) and chewing gum. Forty-two people with moderate to severe periodontal disease and twenty-five people with healthy gums chewed gum fifty times on each side of their mouth. The investigators measured the level of endotoxins before chewing and five to ten minutes after chewing. According to the report, the average amount of endotoxins present in the blood was significantly higher in all the patients after the gum chewing. Those with severe periodontal disease were nearly four times as likely to have significant levels of endotoxins after chewing than those with healthy gums.[6] You can decide whether it is a good idea to chew gum.

Smoking and Free Radicals

Smoking is a major risk factor for periodontitis (inflammation of the gums) and may be responsible for more than half of periodontitis cases among adults in the United States. A large proportion of adult periodontitis may be prevented by not smoking or quitting smoking.[7] Smoking causes free-radical damage to the gums and reduces the vitamins in your entire system, specifically vitamin C.[8] It seems that smoking lowers the antioxidant levels throughout the body and not only causes gingivitis (inflammation of the gums) but also systemic inflammation. This inflammation increases the possibility of all degenerative diseases.[9] The cougher's hack may be more than just annoying to the person who coughs and those nearby, causing inflammation and an overworked immune system to the cougher. The more you smoke, the more advanced the disease can become, and the more free radicals are generated.[10]

PREGNANCY, INFANCY AND CHILDHOOD PROBLEMS

Inflammation does not just affect adults. It can also pose health risks to children during infancy and beyond, as well as during pregnancy, during which time the developing fetus can be saddled with predispositions to the same disease conditions affecting their mothers. Let's examine the factors that can cause inflammation in expectant mothers and their children.

Pregnancy and Pre-Pregnancy

If I could talk all parents who plan to have children into removing junk food and foods to which they are sensitive, they would have much healthier children. Research with rats shows the importance of the fetal environment. For example, restricted protein in pregnant rats has been linked to a higher rate of diabetes in offspring when they mature.[1] Eating from Food Plan II or III (see Chapter 7) for six months before pregnancy, and continuing through delivery provides the best chance of giving birth to a baby with a healthy endocrine system. In addition, your child will likely have fewer allergies, health problems, and congenital defects (conditions present at birth). Of course, exercising and constructively dealing with stress during pregnancy, as well as eliminating allergens, are also required for a healthy child. My Body Monitor Kit (see Chapter 6) is a great and easy test for the harmful effects of all these factors on your health and that of your baby.

Many medical journal articles show that harmful chemicals cause learning disabilities, hyperactivity, and other disorders. These chemicals can damage the delicate brain growth process in the unborn child during pregnancy. A fetus can also be damaged by the following chemicals: pesticides, cigarettes, alcohol, coffee, fluoride, MSG, anesthesia, cosmetics, mercury, perfume fragrance, artificial food additives, vaccines, marijuana, aspirin, damaged sperm, ultrasound, prescription drugs, excessive junk food, and excessive sugar.[2]

Dr. W. H. Wilson investigated why infants had recurring ear infections (otitis media) during the time they were breast-fed. Wilson believes that children acquire immune complexes to certain foods in the womb that reflected the mother's allergies. Wilson determined which foods caused allergies in the mothers and removed the foods from the mother's diet. The nursing infant's ear problems subsequently cleared up.[3] These results suggest that specific allergies and a general tendency for allergies can be passed down through generations. The breastfeeding period can be thought of as a last stage of pregnancy, where the mother's allergies can affect the child through her milk.

Periodontal disease in a pregnant woman can be a risk factor for miscarriage and premature birth, as well. Mouth infections cause inflammation associated with an elevation of prostaglandins and cytokines in the bloodstream. Over-active prostaglandins and cytokines are, by definition, immune responses. One known cause of miscarriages is an immune reaction of the mother's body to the fetus. Overall, studies have concluded that increased risk of miscarriage is anywhere from three to eight times as great when a woman suffers from periodontal disease. A recent study found that the worse the gum disease is, the more likely a woman is to have an early-term birth. One of the researchers suggests that women contemplating pregnancy and those already pregnant should ask their dentist to examine them for periodontal disease.[4] If periodontal disease is found, it should be dealt with immediately. (For more on periodontal disease, see page 101.)

Newborns and Infants

What precautions should parents take to ensure that their newborn grows up healthy? First, breastfeed the infant for as long as possible, ideally, for at least four months. Look into hypoallergenic baby formulas after the baby has been weaned from breast milk, or if the mother cannot nurse. Listed below are other things that all parents, whether they are combating an allergy history, or just trying to strengthen their child's immune system, should do.

- Do not give a baby a formula in the first weeks of life.

- Wait at least six months before feeding beef to a baby.

- Wait at least six months after birth to give cow's milk and make sure the child can tolerate it at that age. I am not sure cow's milk is necessary at any age.

- Do not smoke in the presence of any baby.

- Wait at least two years to put a child in daycare.

The first two years are so important in a child's life. Children cannot grow up with a healthy independency if they have not had a good dependency. The more a mother can be with a child to bond in the first two years, the healthier a child will be in later years. In terms of eating, the first two years are also important. A mother has to be aware of how a child reacts to food and make sure the child is getting the right food. Daycare centers have many children, and some are sick at different times. The immune system is not fully developed at birth. Exposing a baby to too many germs can be difficult on the whole body, especially on the immune system.

It is important for the mother to watch for symptoms of allergy in children. In one study, eczema (atopic dermatitis) was found in newborns (15 to 75 days after birth), who were not exclusively breast-fed. When the mothers removed eggs and cow's milk from their children's diet, the infants' eczema ceased in every case. The researchers concluded that food antigens, via breast milk, can get into the bloodstream of infants, causing adverse symptoms.[5] Dr. George Ulett tested umbilical cord blood in infants before food entered the GI tract and found sensitivities to the same foods to which one of the parents were allergic. Sometimes the predisposition for that allergy is passed on and the allergy only surfaces when the corresponding food is introduced.[6]

Most physicians feel that children outgrow their allergies. I do not agree. Children could outgrow obvious symptoms only to see them manifest in different forms when they become adults, such as changing to arthritis, multiple sclerosis, or other diseases. Dr. D. C. Heiner's research shows that when an adult has a respiratory disease, food allergy should be considered if there was a history of prior intolerance to a food in childhood.[7] My research confirms this, but expands this diagnostic advice to all diseases of unknown origin.

Babies have an increased intestinal permeability to proteins and macromolecules during the first four months after birth. This intestinal leakiness can disappear with the subsequent maturation of the intestinal wall.[8] Some researchers believe that if the wall is not given enough time to mature and the baby is exposed to cow's milk, the milk antigen will get into the bloodstream, causing milk allergy and inflammation. For some it can cause asthma and eczema in childhood and various other problems as adults.[9] Researchers have also found that reactions to milk and wheat during childhood could either trigger autism or worsen neurological symptoms. The authors of the study suggested that the proteins in food caused toxic effects in the central nervous system by interacting with neurotransmitters.[10]

Children

A study determined how many children developed an allergy to cow's milk during the early years of childhood. Researchers monitored thirty-seven children for one to seven years and found the following early symptoms: diarrhea, failure to develop, vomiting, blood in the stools, colic, asthma, and eczema. Towards the end of the study, twelve children still had some of the original symptoms and twenty-seven children (73 percent) developed other symptoms, such as rhinitis, angioedema, and urticaria.[11]

Learning disabilities are on the rise and have also been linked to allergy. In one study many types of synthetic petroleum chemicals and known problem foods were removed from the diet of children who had learning disabilities. As a result, learning abilities improved.

Twenty-one autistic children, who were thought to be otherwise healthy, were tested for intestinal permeability. An altered permeability was found in nine of the twenty-one (43 percent) autistic patients but in none of the forty controls. The researchers speculate that an altered intestinal permeability could represent a possible mechanism for the increased passage of protein through mucosa, causing inflammation and subsequent behavioral abnormalities.[12]

Dr. A. J. Wakefield studied children who had long standing intestinal symptoms consisting of abdominal pain, constipation, diarrhea (or alternating constipation and diarrhea), and bloating. These children had behavioral problems, and their symptoms had often started at around the same time as behavioral changes. The children in the study ate the same foods day after day, with a diet limited largely to cereals, potato chips, and bread. Despite this, they typically seemed well-nourished, with height and weight in the normal limits. Certain foodstuffs, such as dairy products, were reported by parents to produce negative behavior, whereas withholding such foods apparently produced behavioral improvement—in particular, for aggression, eye contact, and normal sleeping. According to parental reports, recognizably undigested food was often seen in stools. That study also confirmed an increase in mucus in the bloodstream and cells.[13]

Children with attention-deficit/hyperactivity disorder (ADHD) are seven times more likely to have food allergies than children in the general population, according to the results of a study headed by Dr. Joseph A. Bellanti. "Food allergy may play a role in the development of ADHD." Bellanti and his colleagues used food allergy tests to assess the presence of food allergies in seventeen children diagnosed with ADHD who ranged in age from 7 to 10 years. Fifty-six percent had positive food allergy tests, compared with six to eight percent positive food allergy tests among children in the general population.[14] This is just one of many medical journal articles that show the relationship between food allergy and ADHD.[15]

The measles, mumps, and rubella (MMR) vaccine may also make infants susceptible to food allergies. A primary effect of the MMR vaccination is the production of interferon gamma, which is known to alter intestinal cells and increase intestinal permeability, causing inflammation.[16] Additionally, the blood-brain barrier becomes more permeable allowing lymphocytes to infiltrate the brain. This can result in serious mental effects such as learning disabilities, behavioral problems, and/or schizophrenia. Researchers are still looking into other related causes of intestinal and blood-brain barrier permeability, like genetics or infections, which might work with the MMR's vaccine production of interferon gamma.[17]

Ileocolonic lymphonodular hyperplasia, a new form of inflammatory bowel disease in children with developmental disorders, has a high correlation to usage of the MMR vaccine. In one study, seventy-five out of ninety-one children who received the vaccine tested positive for the measles virus in their intestinal tissue, compared to five of seventy control subjects.[18] If a child has ADD (attention deficit disorder) or ADHD and has had the MMR vaccine, make sure that all other factors that could be causing the problem are explored and resolved. It is possible that the MMR is continually challenging his or her immune system and removing other substances that challenge the immune system would be a great help in alleviating the problem.

The relationship between the intestinal tract and the brain may also be responsible for some of the behavioral features of autism. This hypothesis was first proposed as early as 1979 by Dr J. Panksepp.[19] It is called the opiod excess hypothesis and has only recently found increasing acceptance in the pediatric psychiatry community. Proteins that have an opiod effect of dietary origin have been identified in the urine of some children with autistic enterocolitis (inflammation in the intestines and colon). These studies certainly show the mind-body connection working overtime.

I found a similar story on the Internet that many of you will identify with:

I have two boys, one with ADD and one with ADHD. The one with ADHD has more severe allergic symptoms than the one diagnosed with ADD. The first one is allergic to dust, mold, tree pollen, grasses, and one medicine so far, Amoxicillen. He is also lactose intolerant. He has a slight hearing problem due to the severity and number of ear infections he suffered when younger. He is now 13. The other has had only the diagnosis of hay fever and is also allergic to Amoxicillen.

As a start, if these boys would remove all sugar, wheat, and dairy from their diet for two weeks, I think the mother would be pleasantly surprised by the positive effects this change could have on their symptoms. Testing these boys for all food allergies would help them tremendously. But many physicians still fail to recognize the link between bad diet, food allergy, and ADD and ADHD.

Much of this research shows that the foods to which one is allergic can be instrumental in causing symptoms and diseases. When children are having behavioral or physical problems make sure that free radicals, AGEs, food allergies, and chemical sensitivities do not contribute to them. Ridding the digestive tract of yeast, parasites, and abnormal bacteria, and replacing the probiotics (see Chapter 7) will help alleviate inflammation and allergies. This will help food that we eat to work at the cellular level. Also make sure that the child is getting all the love possible to enhance his or her ability to digest foods. All of this will help rid the body of a multitude of seemingly unrelated symptoms.

RESPIRATORY DISEASES
Asthma, Chronic Bronchitis, and Emphysema

There are basically two types of respiratory diseases: acute and chronic. Acute respiratory diseases have symptoms such as coughs, colds, bronchitis, and pneumonia. These diseases are mostly due to infections, and are relatively short-lived. Most can be easily curtailed with today's drugs. Chronic conditions, like asthma, bronchitis, and emphysema are more difficult to treat. This section deals with chronic conditions. After investigating the research, I have found that the causes are similar for all chronic respiratory diseases; therefore, they will all be discussed together.

As far back as 1984, Dr. D.C. Heiner's research has shown that respiratory tract symptoms may be exclusively due to food allergy, or may be combined with chemical sensitivity. He also believes that, in *rare* cases, respiratory diseases can be due to a congenital defect of the heart or tracheo-bronchial tree. I agree. A few people are born with a congenital defect that makes them more susceptible to a variety of diseases, including respiratory diseases.[1] Research supports that there are a host of respiratory diseases that are related to food allergy. These include:

- Rhinitis.

- Inflammation in the ear.

- Enlarged tonsillar and adenoid tissues.

- Lower respiratory tract disease such as chronic coughing, wheezing, and bleeding from the mouth.[2]

When food allergy symptoms are involved with the lower respiratory tract, the food allergy reaction is usually delayed, and IgG
blood tests will detect these reactions. Preventing exposure to foods
to which a person reacts at an early age can prevent lung diseases
later on.[3] The food allergy can cause irritation which may lead to
inflammation, increasing the likelihood of asthma and other respiratory diseases.

Air pollution and chemicals can also be a problem in bronchial
conditions.[4] While a person is getting well it is a good idea to isolate
and remove any chemicals to which that person may have an allergic reaction. Also make sure there are no low-grade infections. If
there are, they can be dealt with medically.

Oxidative stress caused by smoking cigarettes induces a chronic
inflammatory response.[5] Anyone with respiratory disease needs to
be no closer than twenty feet to smoke, which means the room they
are in. This inflammation can lead to bronchitis, emphysema, asthma,
and lung cancer. Although smoking causes oxidative stress, research
shows that non-smokers with asthma have increased oxidative stress
as well. One study was performed on twenty-four children being
treated for severe bronchial asthma. The control group consisted of
twenty-seven healthy children. The study revealed that children suffering from bronchial asthma exhibit increased oxidative stress. The
authors support the theory of the involvement of free radicals in
severe bronchial asthma. Other factors such as mold exposure may
act as nonspecific triggers for the development of asthma also.[6]

Although respiratory disease might show symptoms primarily in
the lungs, the whole body can be affected. Some people with respiratory diseases have the following symptoms:

1. Inflammation throughout the body.

2. Nutritional abnormalities and weight loss.

3. Loss of muscular ability, skeletal muscle dysfunction.[7]

This research shows how respiratory disease affects the *whole body*. In order to heal the whole person, it is necessary to take a holistic approach to health. In Part Three, you will find more solutions for doing so.

RHEUMATIC DISEASES

Behcet's Disease, Bursitis, Fibromyalgia, Gout, Juvenile Rheumatoid Arthritis, Osteoarthritis (OA), Polyarteritis Nodosa, Polymyalgia Rheumatica, Psoriatic Arthritis, Relapsing Polychondritis, Rheumatoid Arthritis (RA), Scleroderma (Systemic Sclerosis), Sjögren's Syndrome, Spondyloarthropathies (Common-form Ankylosing Spondylitis), Systemic Lupus Erythematosus, Temporal Arteritis, Tendinitis, and Wegener's Granulomatosis

Inflammation that damages joints and connective tissue is known as rheumatic disease. Debate has persisted for some time as to whether the causes are purely internal, in which the body turns on itself (autoimmune disease), or if there are other causes. I have never been convinced that ailments happen in the absence of contributing lifestyle factors. Something from our environment, including the foods we eat, induces inflammation, causing these diseases.

Rheumatoid Arthritis (RA)

Rheumatoid arthritis (RA), an extremely common inflammatory disease of the synovium (joint lining), strikes hands, wrists, elbows, shoulders, and knees. The disease can also cause widespread inflammation in blood vessels throughout the body, putting a person at risk for heart disease and other diseases. Research shows that RA can double a woman's risk of suffering a heart attack. If a woman has rheumatoid arthritis for at least a decade, her risk for having a heart attack triples. Some of the cells that can be found in inflamed joints also turn up in the plaques that develop inside artery linings.[1] Once you upset your body chemistry and homeostasis can no longer be maintained, one problem leads to the next.

Research shows that people with arthritis have elevated levels of C-reactive protein (CRP).[2] It could be from AGEs, infections, smoking, or food and chemical sensitivities. As far back as 1980, there has been research showing the relationship between food allergy and arthritis.[3] Unfortunately not many people took these findings seriously. Dr. Carinini and Dr. Brostroff studied food-induced arthritis. They stated:

> Despite an increasing interest in food allergy and the conviction of innumerable patients with joint disease that certain foods exacerbate their symptoms, relatively little scientific attention has been paid to this relationship. Abnormalities of the gastrointestinal tract are commonly found in rheumatic disease. Support for an intestinal origin of antigens comes from studies of patients whose joint symptoms have improved on the avoidance of certain foods antigens, and become worse on consuming them.[4]

Researchers believe that food allergy applies to people with intermittent symptoms, as well as acute and chronic arthritis. Arthritic people can react to any food and do so according to their individual genetic blueprint. See page 26 for a list of the most common food allergies.

Many people with arthritis react to gluten products. Dr. C. Little's studies show that serotonin became elevated in the bloodstream after the ingestion of gluten in sensitive people.[5] Dr. A. Parks also researched food allergy and arthritis, drawing the same conclusions as Little. Parks went on to show the allergic mechanism that causes rheumatoid arthritis—the same process that was discussed in Chapter 2.

> The gastrointestinal tract must be permeable to the gluten proteins, derived from the digested gluten. This digested protein (food antigen) appears in the bloodstream and binds with an antibody (probably IgG or IgA, not IgE). The antigen and antibody form a circulating immune complex (CIC). The CICs activate the rest of the immune response. Serotonin is one of the chemicals. This causes the symptoms of arthritis. As serotonin circulates in the bloodstream, the CICs deposit in joint tissues. There they activate complement, which in turn damages cells and activates more inflammation. More inflammation results in more pain, swelling, stiffness, and loss of mobility.[6]

Two studies led researchers to the conclusion that drinking decaffeinated coffee is a risk factor in rheumatoid arthritis. In one study, women who drank four or more cups of decaffeinated coffee a day had more than twice the risk of developing RA. In a similar study, researchers evaluated risk factors for developing rheumatoid arthritis among 64,000 black women who were followed from 1995 to 2000 as part of the Black Women's Health Study. Among the sampled women, those who drank more than one cup of decaffeinated coffee a day seemed to quadruple their risk of developing rheumatoid arthritis. However, regular coffee brought no increased risk, and three cups a day or more of tea reduced the risk of the disease by 60 percent, leading to speculation that industrial solvents in decaffeinated coffee may play a role in the arthritic process.[7] Unfortunately, the researchers did not consider the amount of sugar these women were consuming in their tea, coffee, or in other products, nor how many allergy-inducing foods they were eating each day. More of these patients would have been symptom-free if the researchers had them tested for other food reactions and removed the sugar.

Other scientists have found that milk allergy can trigger arthritis.[8] Remember that any food can trigger an allergic reaction, and most of the time more than one food triggers arthritic symptoms.[9] All foods that a person eats on a regular basis should be considered as possible allergens.

Osteoarthritis (OA)

Affecting an estimated 21 million adults in the U.S., osteoarthritis (OA) primarily affects cartilage, the tissue that cushions the ends of bones within the joint. The frayed or non-existent cartilage leads to inflammation, joint pain, and stiffness. Disability results most often when the disease affects the spine and the weight-bearing joints (knees and hips). Pain in the early morning upon awakening, and pain and stiffness while standing up after sitting in one position for an extended period of time are some of the early signs of osteoarthritis. As some people age, there is increased formation of AGEs, which result in increased cross-linking of the cartilage matrix, causing stiffness and activation of cytokines. Although this is commonly thought to happen with age, I do not think it necessarily happens if you keep your body in homeostasis as you get older.

One study showed that wheat, nuts, spices, corn, tomatoes, bell peppers, potatoes, salt, iodine containing foods (onions, turnips, sea weeds), string beans, chocolate, fish, citrus fruits, cheese, milk, yams, peaches, pears, and artichokes all caused OA symptoms.[10] A food allergy test will help you find out if the foods you eat are affecting you.

Although osteoarthritis has been called "wear and tear" disease, I do not believe this. There are many older people who have been avid runners for many years who do not have osteoarthritis. The pain might become exacerbated when you run, but running or other exercise does not cause it. The Tarahumara Indians who inhabit mountains in Mexico have a long life span. They are known to be avid runners all their lives, but don't have any forms of arthritis. Remember that these native people eat an indigenous diet, avoiding processed foods. Unfortunately, the native Indians of Mexico are gradually beginning to adopt the lifestyle of modern civilization, and the processed foods that come with it. There is no doubt that arthritis and other degenerative diseases will take hold in their villages soon.

Juvenile Rheumatoid Arthritis

Juvenile rheumatoid arthritis is the most common form of arthritis in childhood, causing pain, stiffness, swelling, and loss of joint function. It can also be associated with rashes or fevers, affecting various parts of the body. Research into juvenile rheumatoid arthritis has been limited, though one study showed a relationship between juvenile rheumatoid arthritis and milk.[11] Since the symptoms of this childhood arthritis are similar to RA, the same treatment should apply. I believe that children with this disease should explore all potential causes, including food allergy.

Fibromyalgia

Fibromyalgia is a chronic disorder that causes pain throughout the tissues that support and move the bones and joints. Pain, stiffness, and localized tender points occur in the muscles and tendons, particularly those of the neck, spine, shoulders, and hips. Patients may also experience fatigue and sleep disturbances. Since the onset of most viral infections and many other well-known diseases begin with aching, fatigue, and changes in cognitive dysfunction, it is important to test for bacterial and viral infection and treat them if necessary.[12]

For some people, some of the first signs of fibromyalgia are gastrointestinal problems, a sign of food allergy, and possibly a delayed reaction. Although any food might be the cause, common foods such as milk, wheat, eggs, meat, and coffee have been known to cause symptoms.[13] Fibromyalgia's leading symptoms are migraine, depression, joint pain, and asthma. Since many who suffer with fibromyalgia are frail, it is important to find all inhalants and chemicals—such as cigarette smoke, perfume, and fresh paint—in their environment that might exacerbate the disorder, and remove them. However, do not neglect food allergy testing.[14]

Dr. Kelly Krohn cites more symptoms associated with fibromyalgia that can affect all tissues, organs, and glands.

- Abdominal pain—most often due to irritable bowel syndrome.

- Numbness and tingling in the extremities.

- Cold intolerance—often associated with Raynaud's phenomenon (chronic constriction and spasm of the blood vessels in the fingers, toes, ears, and tip of nose).

- Urinary frequency and urgency—irritable bladder.

- Restless legs.

- Sleep apnea (temporary stoppage of breathing during sleep), more common in men with fibromyalgia.

- Growth hormone deficiency.

- Psychological stress.

- Sicca symptoms (dry eyes and dry mouth).[15]

People with fibromyalgia have an immune system that is unable to mitigate these symptoms. If a load can be taken off of the immune system, the body has a better chance to heal. All causes should be taken into account including the psychological.

Systemic Lupus Erythematosus (SLE), Lupus, Lupus Erythematosus (LE)

Systemic lupus erythematosus (SLE) is an autoimmune disease in which the immune system harms the body's own healthy cells and tissues. The result is inflammation of, and damage to, the joints, skin, kidneys, heart, lungs, blood vessels, and brain. Potential antigens that cause the damage include pollens, chemicals, foods, medications, and germs.

Dr. A.C. Brown did extensive research of the scientific literature from 1950 to 2000 on SLE and its relationship to nutrition.[16] He found that foods can aggravate the symptoms. So can excess calories (eating too much), excess protein, high fat (especially saturated and omega-6 polyunsaturated fatty acids), zinc, iron, and L-canavanine (found in alfalfa tablets).

Some people with systemic SLE, when placed on food allergy elimination diets, reported improvement in their symptoms.[17] Sometimes a person goes into remission for unknown reasons. When a person is in remission, the pain is less. Without knowing it, these people consumed less allergy inducing foods and decreased the load on their immune systems and whole bodies.

Israeli researchers determined that 56 percent of lupus patients had an allergy, compared to 10 percent of the general population, and 21 percent had two allergies. The most common symptom was dermatosis (a skin disorder), due to the consumption of food (51 percent) or drugs (31 percent), compared to 11 percent and 5 percent of the incidence of the control group, respectively. In addition, other allergies were also more prevalent in SLE patients. Conjunctivitis (inflammation of the clear membrane that coats the inner lining of the eyelids and the outer surface of the eye) was present in 26 percent (control group: 9 percent), and rhinitis was present in 34 percent (control group: 13 percent). Finally, asthma was present in 47 percent of the SLE patients and only in 6 percent of the control group. Dr. Vera Machtelincks found that patients with SLE are frequently bothered with allergies and that both diseases are based on certain similar pathogenic mechanisms. In the study it was noted that children of mothers with SLE often had more allergies than expected.[18] There is no doubt in my mind that SLE patients could be helped with food allergy testing.

Other Contributing Factors to Rheumatic Disease

Rheumatic diseases can also be caused or exacerbated by nightshade vegetables, stress, AGEs and free radicals.

Nightshade Plants

People with rheumatoid symptoms should try eliminating night-shade vegetables, including white potatoes, red and green peppers, tomatoes, pimiento, cayenne, eggplant, and tobacco. These plants contain solanine, which can be toxic if not destroyed in the intestine. Research shows that many people were helped by removing night-shade plants, but I have not found this in my practice. I believe that a person might be allergic to one or more but not necessarily all the nightshade plants. You have nothing to lose, so remove them all for two weeks and see what happens.

If solanine removal is found to help, remove all tomatoes and peppers from your diet, and make sure you check for nightshade plants that could be hidden in soups, salads, and casseroles. It may take up to six months to get results with this approach. However, in two surveys, 28 percent and 44 percent of people, respectively, had "marked positive responses when nightshade vegetables were eliminated from their diet."[19] It might be more effective to test for all allergies and remove all foods to which you react. This way healing is much faster.

Stress

Dr. A.J. Zautra and associates provided support for the proposition that emotional turmoil can increase arthritis. In one study depression affected both RA and OA patients.[20] In another study of working conditions, the psycho-social environment of the workplace contributed to arthritic symptoms.[21] Letting the stress in your life become distress can be another stimulus to create arthritic pain.

AGEs and Free Radicals

Levels of glycation can also affect the progression of disease in patients with OA and RA. "Progressive destruction of arterial cartilage is a hallmark of osteoarthritis and rheumatoid arthritis," say investigators from the Gaubius Laboratory in Leiden, Netherlands.[22] AGEs are an inevitable process in living, but can be accelerated under such pathological conditions as oxidative stress. The two stressors, oxidative stress and glycation stress, can go hand in hand. Raised AGE levels have been found in the serum and synovial fluid of patients with RA.[23] So many people have been helped from removing foods to which they react that I feel that allergies are one of the first things to explore in all joint and connective tissue diseases. Make sure your diet does not increase AGEs or free radicals.

Other conditions can cause arthritis and all must be explored. These include intestinal pathogens like *Shigella, campylobacter,* and *Klebsiella* (all bacteria); and yeast (*Candida albicans*) in the gastrointestinal system, caused by antibiotics, oral contraceptives, steroid medications, and an increased use of alcohol and/or sugar. Treatment of *Candida* infections in the digestive system has improved rheumatoid symptoms in many cases. One often induces these symptoms through his or her own actions without knowing it. Become the detective and try to figure out what you are doing to cause your symptoms and disease.

SURGERY PROBLEMS

Surgical inflammation has also been called surgical stress and can be caused or heightened by the age and health of a given patient, medications, blood transfusions, and psychological stress felt by the patient. Other factors which can cause surgical stress are tissue injury, redistribution of blood flow in the blood vessels, organs being stressed by the surgical procedure, and possible complications, before, during, and after surgery.[1] It is difficult to distinguish as to what stress causes the inflammation. Anesthesia can also trigger inflammation, though it inhibits the effects of surgery by reducing pain and helping to maintain homeostasis during the procedure.[2]

Basically, the inflammatory response to anesthesia and surgery is a beneficial reaction. It is needed for wound healing and for preventing the body from making antibodies against its own tissues. During uncomplicated conventional surgery, the immune response is a healthy one without any harmful effects. When the immune system does not respond or responds erratically, however, there can be harm to the patient. Negative responses may contribute to the development of postoperative infections and the spread of malignant disease.[3] The inflammation can be specific to the site of the surgery, or it can spread to the entire body. Many of the white blood cells are involved in this response to initiate or enhance inflammation.

Transplants

Transplants can cause complications when the immune system rejects the newly transplanted organ. Even when the organ is not rejected, inflammation can be intense. CRP is the blood test that monitors inflammation after surgery and shows if the transplant person is at risk of severe transplant-related complications and mortality.[4]

A problem with allergies has become evident for organ donors and recipients. A new precedent may need to be set for future organ donors, according to a report in the *Archives of Internal Medicine.* Organ donors may need to be screened for allergies to prevent IgE antibodies from being transferred from the donor to the recipient. In one example, a man received a liver transplant from a donor who had died of an anaphylactic reaction to peanuts after a history of allergies. After recovering from the anaphylactic reaction, the transplant patient underwent a skin prick test that was positive for peanuts, cashew nuts, and sesame seeds. The donor had IgE specific antibodies for these same three foods.

This case illustrates that organ donors should be screened for allergies since IgE allergens can be transferred with a liver transplantation. Possibly IgG allergy can also be transferred. Organ recipients should also be aware of the potential dangers and be informed about allergen avoidance.[5]

Recipients of transplanted organs face many problems. Hopefully the information in this book will reduce the number of transplants that are necessary. If one is necessary, this information might help a transplant patient in future years.

* * *

CONCLUSION

There are many, many other diseases that can be dealt with by removing food allergies, chemical sensitivities, AGEs, free radicals, and distress. Some of these diseases are: pancreatitis,[1] eye inflammation,[2] gallbladder disease,[3] liver disease,[4] and PMS (premenstrual syndrome).[5] I believe that when all the research is in, inflammation will be the root of all diseases; therefore, all diseases will be treated in a similar way.

Throughout this section I covered specific diseases, explaining their causes and showing you how to stop causing the inflammation associated with them. In Part Three, I will explain various tests for inflammation and provide you with general guidelines for keeping your body healthy so you can prevent inflammation in the first place.

PART THREE

Guidelines for Preventing and Reversing Inflammation

6

Testing for Inflammation and Other Risk Factors

I n order to most effectively reduce your risk of inflammation, it is important that you be tested for it, as well as for the risk factors associated with it, which we discussed in Part One (see Chapters 3 and 4). Many people affected by inflammation and these risk factors are unaware that they are until it is too late. For example, more than a third of all heart attacks directly related to inflammation occur without warning or any preceding, noticeable symptoms. Such incidents could be prevented if the inflammation were detected beforehand.

Doctors have a battery of tests at their disposal that cover almost every chemical reaction and process in the body. In this chapter, I focus on the tests that best detect and quantify levels of inflammation, as well as those you can use to determine if you are affected by infections, AGEs, free radicals and oxidative stress, food and airborne allergies, and heavy metals. Also included are tests to help determine your body's level of homeostasis. These tests can only obtained through a health care practitioner, and as a preventive measure, I recommend that you schedule an annual appointment to have them done. I have not given a reference range for these tests because different labs use different reference ranges and some health care professionals have their own optimal range. Make sure you get and keep a copy of all the laboratory reports that you receive. Then, if necessary, you can have these reports with you should you decide to get a second opinion or to consult a specialist. I suggest that, if any of your blood tests are out of the normal range and you are not comfortable with the practitioner's ideas of how to deal with the situation, you

get the advice of another practitioner. Remember, you are in charge
of your health, not a practitioner.

TESTS FOR INFLAMMATION

Every blood laboratory tests for C-reactive protein (CRP), an indicator of generalized inflammation in the blood. If the results indicate
high levels of CRP, further tests or observation (such as for periodontal disease—See Chapter 5) can help localize the inflammation
and determine the cause, although sometimes the inflammation is
difficult to find. Inflammation can be a part of a natural process or an
unnatural process, so a health practitioner's advice should be
sought.[1] When getting the results from this test, make sure you get
an actual quantitative number, not just a simple result of positive or
negative. If the test just shows a positive reading, you will not know
how extensive the inflammation is, whereas, with a quantitative
number, your results will be more meaningful.

If your test result reveals elevated levels of CRP, there are other
tests your doctor can order to attempt to learn more about the degree
of inflammation you suffer from. These more specific tests for inflammation include:

Homocysteine: to determine if you are at high risk of a heart
attack or stroke. This test can also be used to determine if you suffer
from folate or vitamin B_{12} deficiency, as homocysteine levels can be
elevated when either deficiency is present.

Interleukin 2: measures your body's ability to fight off infectious
invaders that can also cause inflammation to occur.

Interleukin 6: used in diagnosing heart disease, the initial signs
of which might otherwise go undetected.

Tumor necrosis factor: although used primarily to diagnose
rheumatoid arthritis, this test can also be used to screen for elevated
levels of endotoxins from bacteria that are often present in many
cases of inflammatory disease.

Lipoprotein A: used to determine if you are at high risk for heart
disease.

Cytokines (proteins secreted during the inflammatory process):
used to assess cellular responses to various endotoxins, including
antigens and bacteria.

Eukotrienes: used to detect the presence of inflammatory compounds that have strong actions on many essential organs and

systems, including the cardiovascular, pulmonary, and central nervous system, as well as the gastrointestinal tract and the immune system.

Sed rate: (erythrocyte sedimentation rate; ESR) usually used to test for rheumatoid arthritis, this test can also be used to monitor inflammation, malignant disease, rheumatic fever, tuberculosis, and heart attack.

Fibrinogen: used primarily to measure the concentration of fibrinogen in the blood, this test can also be used to evaluate abnormal blood clotting.

Histamine: used to detect states of altered reactivity in which the body reacts with an exaggerated immune response to a foreign substance, indicating allergy.

Eosinophils: used to screen for parasitic organisms, as well as for allergic reactions.

TESTS FOR INFECTIONS

There are two basic blood tests. They are a complete blood count (CBC) and blood chemistry 25 or 21.

Complete Blood Count (CBC): provides a good profile of your red blood cells and your white blood cells, thus also providing a good indication of the health of your immune system.

Blood Chemistry 25 and 21: determine the status of other items of basic importance in your bloodstream, such as your blood glucose, cholesterol, triglycerides, calcium, blood urea nitrogen and others.

These tests can reveal the presence of infections, but what they do even better is reveal imbalances in the body chemistry, providing a snapshot of your overall homeostasis. If the tests detect factors out of the normal range, other tests can be given to get more specific information about the imbalances that are found.

TESTS FOR *CANDIDA ALBICANS*

In addition to the CBC and blood chemistry tests, for many people testing for *Candida Albicans*, an overgrowth of fungus, can also be important. The most common tests used for this purpose are:

The *Candida* Immune Complex Assay Test: this blood test detects the presence of antibodies that fight off yeast infections. If antibodies are present, usually this means *Candida* is too.

Stool Test: an exam of stool under a microscope may reveal the presence of *Candida*.

***Candida* culture:** if one of the symptoms is oral thrush (a white coating on the tongue), a culture may be taken from the tongue.

TEST FOR AGEs

The most common test for AGEs is known as the hemoglobin A1c (glycosylated hemoglobin) blood test. This test measures the amount of sugars that are attached non-enzymatically to your body's proteins. It also shows your blood glucose control over a six-to eight-week period, enabling physicians to determine whether AGEs have advanced in the body.

TEST FOR FREE-RADICAL DAMAGE AND OXIDATIVE STRESS

A urine test for glutathione (GSH) and blood lipid peroxides will enable you to determine the level of stress on your body caused by free-radical damage. The GSH level provides a direct measure of the amount of free-radical damage in the body, indicating the liver's potential for breaking down drugs and eliminating toxic by-products. An elevated serum peroxide level indicates the amount of lipids damaged by oxidants, which is a reflection of excessive free radical activity. Other tests for free radical damage and oxidative stress include sodium oxide dismutase (SOD), gluthathione peroxidase, and hydroxyl radical markers, all of which also provide indications of the degree that free-radical damage is causing stress in the body.

The oxidative stress indicator (OSI) is a simple breath test that focuses on the breakdown of fatty acids, most commonly found in oily fish and flaxseed oil. Ethane forms when oxygenated free radicals destroy fatty acids. The OSI test shows how far free radicals have progressed. Deficiencies of these fatty acids are strongly linked to heart disease and depression, and may also play a part in other neuro-developmental conditions. The test makes it easier to determine if enough antioxidants are being consumed in the diet, and whether or not they are being destroyed due to food allergy, distress, or other factors. This is an excellent test to help prevent dangerous levels of oxidative stress from occurring. The OSI, designed as an easy to use home-testing kit, is particularly ideal for use with children. The breath test can be performed in the comfort of your own home, or, if preferred, through a healthcare professional.

ALLERGY TESTING

All people with chronic and degenerative diseases should be tested for food and airborne allergies. Both blood testing for IgE (immediate reaction) and IgG (delayed reaction) are important. The IgE tests determine the presence of IgE antibody directed to particular foods or airborne potential allergies, while the IgG tests determine the presence of IgG antibody. The symptoms of an IgG reaction are usually delayed from two hours up to two days. On page 20 there is a list of symptoms which can occur with either an IgE or IgG reaction. There are two basic tests to show the presence of IgE antibodies—RAST and the skin prick test, while the IgG ELISA and Prime tests are the most commonly used test to determine the presence of an IgG reaction.

RAST: a blood test used to determine the amount of IgE antibodies to the specific foods suspected of causing allergic reactions. It requires a small blood sample that is sent to a lab that performs the test shortly upon receiving the blood. The level of IgE present does not always correlate to the severity of the allergic reaction.

Skin prick test: performed by exposing a tiny area of scratched skin to the food or foods being evaluated. This is accomplished either by pricking the skin with a small needle or probe through a drop of the food extract, or by using a pricking device that has been pre-soaked in the extract. A positive skin test results in a mosquito-bite-like reaction at the site of the test within minutes. Neither the size of the skin test reaction, nor the level of specific IgE antibody in the blood test, necessarily correlates with the type or severity of allergy symptoms. Consider an allergy evaluation with a positive skin test and a positive RAST test to peanuts. One person with these results may be eating peanuts every day without symptoms, while a different person may experience anaphylaxis from peanuts. Similarly, that second person may experience only an itchy mouth on one occasion, anaphylaxis on another, and a mild case of hives on yet another occasion of peanut exposure.

IgG ELISA: The ELISA (enzyme-linked immunoserological assay) tests the antigen/antibody reaction to determine delayed food reactions (those occurring more than twenty-four hours after the ingestion of foods that trigger an allergic reaction). It requires a small blood sample that is sent to a lab that performs the test within seventy-two hours after the blood is drawn. A computer then analyzes the blood sample, measuring the presence of specific foods and their specific IgG antibodies found in the blood.

Prime Test: This IgG test reveals the damage or death done to white blood cells and other blood components by foods that cause an allergic reaction. It also requires a small blood sample that is sent to a lab that performs the test shortly after the blood is drawn.

These are the basic tests for food allergy. Different medical laboratories call the blood tests by different names, but basically they are similar tests. My experience has been that the RAST and the ELISA blood tests are the most valid, not the skin prick test. For many people, the IgG ELISA and Prime tests are the most important ones, as they screen for hidden allergies that are usually delayed and cause the degenerative diseases. Two other tests that are less expensive and can be useful for many people who do not have lots of allergies are the elimination and challenge diet and the Body Monitor Kit.

Elimination and challenge diet: To perform this test, you will need to abstain from the food group to which you suspect you might be allergic or sensitive, such as all milk and milk products (cheese, cottage cheese, yogurt, ice cream, cream, and kefir) for ten days. After ten days, perform the challenge test by drinking a glass of milk, watching for signs of reaction. Any of the symptoms found on page 20 might be felt or seen. When performing an elimination diet, it is most effective to avoid other foods in the same food family during the test period. When testing for wheat, also remove kamut, spelt (both are wheat), and rye (a first cousin to wheat).

The Body Monitor Kit: This kit can be used easily in your own home to test for food allergies and homeostasis. The advantage of this kit is that you can do it over and over and get a thumbnail sketch of what is going on in your body at that moment. A blood test just tests once. The Body Monitor Kit gets your attention. See page 212 for more details.

When you find the food to which you react, remove it completely for two months. At that time, reintroduce the food, but you must test it twice. Sometimes the body does not set up a reaction until the second eating. Watch for a reaction. If you have one, that food is still not safe to eat. You will be able to reintroduce many foods back into your diet at that time, but not all. A better way to find out if the allergy has been eliminated is to use the Body Monitor Kit to find out if you can reintroduce foods. In an act of perversity for which the cosmos has become famous, people are often sensitive to their favorite foods, particularly those eaten most frequently. So test those foods first.

Some researchers say that more widespread recognition of food allergy would be cost effective for insurance companies, doctors, and patients. Dealing effectively with allergies is a cheap way to get healthy. If you suspect that you have food allergies, ask your health care practitioner about these tests.

Airborne Allergies

Both the skin prick/scratch test and the IgE RAST test can also be used to test for airborne allergies, which are primarily caused by grasses, weeds, molds, and mildew. When the skin prick or scratch test is used, a small amount of an allergy-causing substance is placed on the skin and then there is scratching or pricking of the skin so that the allergen is introduced under the skin surface. A reaction will include swelling and redness of the site. Several substances can be tested at the same time and results are usually obtained within twenty minutes. In the case of the IgE RAST test, the amount of IgE antibody to the specific airborne substance will be measured.

When it comes to airborne allergies, I must emphasize not to have these tests done until you have first removed foods to which you react for two months. The immune system becomes strong enough to deal with the airborne substances that have given you symptoms once you have removed foods to which you react. If you have airborne allergies, whether you know it or not, you have food allergies. Deal with those first.

Tests for Toxic Metals

Elements such as aluminum, arsenic, cadmium, mercury, lead, and copper have been highly correlated with inflammation and disease. Nutrients such as iron, manganese, and selenium can also become toxic when present at excessively high levels in the body. Radiation poisoning, from medical and dental x-rays, building materials, cellular phones, electronic games, microwave ovens and air pollution, can also upset the body chemistry and cause inflammation. There are laboratories that test for individual metal toxicity. Panels of different metals can also be tested, as can radiation toxicity. Your health care practitioner has information on these tests. For more information about what you can do to detoxify from these types of toxins, see Chapter 8.

7

Food Plans and Lifestyle Considerations

Throughout this book, I have repeatedly stressed that our twenty-first century lifestyle, filled as it is with junk food, foods to which our body has become allergic/addicted to, chemicals, and strong emotional tides, is a primary cause of inflammation leading to the many diseases with which we are faced. As we saw in Chapter 2, inflammation occurs only when the body becomes unable to maintain its balance, or homeostasis. The three most important threats to homeostasis are poor diet, unhealthy lifestyle choices, and the buildup of toxins in the body. This chapter provides you with the most effective dietary and lifestyle choices you can take to prevent inflammation altogether, and to reverse it if it has already taken hold of your body, while Chapter 8 provides you with the information you need to safely detoxify yourself.

Based on my 29 years of researching health, as well as my own long-term recovery from chronic illness that began when I was 40—today, at 69, I am much healthier than I was at 21, and also blessed with far more energy—I believe the single most important step you can take to resolve not only inflammation, but any health problem, is to eat a healthy diet and follow a health-promoting lifestyle. Your health is the direct result of what you put in your mouth, and what you *don't* put in your mouth, and how you live your life. In both cases, the choices you make determine how healthy you are. The good news is that you have complete control over both factors.

In this chapter you will learn how to achieve that control using the same food plans and lifestyle guidelines that have helped so many of my readers.

EATING HEALTHY

By choosing to eat healthy foods and eliminating all foods that are harmful to you, you can dramatically improve your health and ensure that inflammation will not affect you. I have seen this time after time with the hundreds of people who consult with me. In every single case, when they improved their diet, they improved their health. Based on such results, I have developed the following food plans, which are effective in helping one achieve and maintain homeostasis and, in turn, reverse inflammation. Choose the plan that is best suited to your current health status. If you are experiencing symptoms such as headaches, allergies, joint pains, general fatigue (especially after meals), or high blood pressure, or if you have a degenerative disease, I recommend that you start out by following Food Plan I. If your symptoms are still present after a week, or if you are still unable to maintain homeostasis (as determined by the Body Chemistry Test), Food Plan II, which is more restrictive, can be tried. If your symptoms still persist, go on to Food Plan III.

Following the food plans may initiate withdrawal symptoms from the addictive foods that are no longer in your diet. Omitting these foods can result in such painful symptoms as fever, depression, headaches, chills, anger, and fatigue. In some people, symptoms may last two or three days; for others, the symptoms may last a week. Please don't be alarmed by such symptoms. They are temporary, and after they pass, you will soon start to notice the health benefits you are looking for. The key to your success lies in committing to the food plan that is most appropriate for you. The guidelines for each food plan are as follows:

Food Plan I

1. Avoid all foods in categories IV and V (see food lists starting on page 134). Eat any other food.

2. If your body is not beginning to feel better after being on Food Plan I for seven days, your body chemistry may require a more stringent food plan. Therefore, proceed with Food Plan II.

Food Plan II

1. Avoid all foods in Categories III, IV, and V (see food lists starting on page 134). For meals, eat foods found in Category I. Foods in Category II may be eaten in small amounts and only between meals.

2. If your symptoms persist after being on Food Plan II for seven days, an even more restrictive plan is needed. If this is the case, proceed with Food Plan III.

Food Plan III

Food Plan III addresses an unbalanced body chemistry involving more than just the foods that are common to body chemistry upset. Food Plan III is designed to provide complete nutrients to your body in their most bio-available form. Foods in this plan are the ones most people can digest, metabolize, and assimilate easily. The procedures and foods of Food Plan III are the least stressful to the body chemistry.

1. For fourteen days, eat only those foods from Category I (see food lists starting on page 134). Eat one small portion from each food group four or five times a day. Remember to also follow the Health-Promoting Eating Habits beginning on page 140.

2. If, after fourteen days, there is no relief of your symptoms and all four arenas have been addressed, a qualified health practitioner can test your blood for food sensitivities. A person in this condition must find foods that do not upset the body chemistry. Choose foods from the following categories according to Food Plans I, II and III.

FOOD CATEGORIES

CATEGORY I

When properly prepared and eaten, these are the foods that are best tolerated by people who have an unbalanced body chemistry.

Green Leafy Vegetables

| Artichoke | Cabbage | Lettuce (all) |
| Brussels sprouts | Kale | Spinach |

Green Vegetables

Alfalfa	Broccoli	Chinese pea pods
Asparagus	Celery	Okra
Avocado*		

*Although avocado is a fruit, it is included in Category I foods.

Root Vegetables

Jicama	Potato	Rutabaga
Onion	Radish	Turnip
Parsnip		

Yellow/White Vegetables

| Cauliflower | Cucumber | Squash (all) |
| Corn | | |

Orange/Purple/Red Vegetables

| Beet | Eggplant | Sweet potato |
| Carrot | Pumpkin | Tomato |

Herbs/Condiments

Arrowroot	Garlic	Parsley
Basil	Ginger	Rosehips
Bay leaf	Horseradish	Rosemary
Black pepper	Lemon	Safflower oil
Butter	Lime	Sage
Caraway	Mustard	Sesame oil

Chili pepper	Nutmeg	Sunflower oil
Chive	Olive oil	Tarragon
Cilantro	Oregano	Thyme
Dill		

Fish

Anchovy	Halibut	Shark
Bass	Mackerel	Shrimp
Catfish	Oyster	Sole
Clam	Perch	Swordfish
Cod	Red snapper	Trout
Crab	Salmon	Tuna
Flounder	Sardine	Any other
Haddock	Scallop	fish

Meats/Poultry*

Bacon	Duck	Pheasant
Beef	Lamb	Pork
Chicken	Liver (beef and	Turkey
Chicken eggs	chicken)	Venison

Beans/Grains

Adzuki beans	Green peas	Red beans
Barley	Kidney beans	Rice, brown (preferred)
Bean sprouts	Lentils	Rice, white
Black beans	Lima beans	Rice, wild
Black-eyed peas	Millet	Rye
Buckwheat	Navy beans	Soybeans
Garbanzo beans	Oats	Split peas
Green beans	Pinto beans	White beans

*If possible eat meat and poultry from free-range, organically fed animals.

Vegetarians can eliminate foods from the Fish and the Meats/Poultry categories and combine the beans and grains for complete protein.

CATEGORY II

Some body chemistries are sensitive to these otherwise wholesome foods:

Fruits

Apples	Figs	Peaches
Apricots	Grapes	Pears
Bananas	Guava	Pineapples
Cantaloupe	Melons (all)	Raspberries
Coconut	Nectarines	Strawberries
Cranberries	Papayas	Watermelon
Dates		

Nuts/Seeds

Almonds	Hickory nuts	Poppy seeds
Brazil nuts	Macadamia nuts	Safflower seeds
Chestnuts	Pecans	Sunflower seeds
Hazelnuts	Pistachios	Walnuts

Herbs/Condiments

Anise seeds	Cream of tartar	Spearmint
Chicory	Paprika	Stevia
Clove		

CATEGORY III

Overcooking, overeating, and eating foods with sugar have turned these normally well-tolerated foods into potentially abusive ones in some people. This includes those who have already compromised their body systems through continued abuse.

Grains

Wheat bran	White flour	Kamut
Wheat germ	Whole wheat	Spelt

Dairy

Buttermilk	Cream cheese	Whey

| Cheese (all) | Milk, cow's | Yogurt |

Fungi

| Mushrooms | Yeast, baker's | Yeast, brewer's |

Fruits

| Grapefruit | Orange | Tangerine |
| Mango | | |

Nuts/Seeds

| Cashews | Peanuts |

Miscellaneous

Carob	Corn gluten	Peppermint
Cinnamon	Cornstarch	Processed foods
Coffee, decaffeinated	Curry	Salt
Coffee, regular	Hops	Tea
Cola bean	Molasses	Vanilla

CATEGORY IV

The following items are always abusive to human body chemistry. Only those who remain adaptive can rebalance after frequent exposure to the items listed here. The more Category IV foods you consume, the more rapid will be the deterioration that occurs in your body chemistry.

Alcohol	Cocoa	Malt
Aspartame	Corn sugar	Maple sugar
Barley malt	Corn syrup	Rice sugar
Beet sugar	Fructose	Saccharin
Cane sugar	Honey	Sucrolose

CATEGORY V

The following substances have been proven to unbalance the body chemistry. It serves good health to stay away from these items or to use them sparingly and with caution. Some of these are used as

The Three-Day Carrot and Green Juice Diet

The Carrot and Green Juice Fast can be done one, two, or three days a month. If you are on any drugs, hypoglycemic or diabetic, or have any serious health condition, consult a physician before you start. Before beginning this fast, follow Food Plan III, (see page 133) for a week. This will start a process of detoxification because you will have eliminated many foods that have made you toxic. You might go through withdrawal symptoms during this week.

A week or more after being on Food Plan III, start a three-day carrot and green juice diet. This will continue the detoxification of your liver, gall bladder, blood and digestive system. It will give your whole body a chance to rest. During the fasting time, you might experience withdrawal symptoms, such as headaches, fatigue, perspiration, depression, shaking, cold body temperature, and general malaise. These symptoms usually will not last for more than two days. When the withdrawal is over, you should feel much better because many of the toxins will have left your body.

If you have a juicer, you can juice the carrots and green vegetables fresh each day. You can use any green vegetables that you like. You might start with celery, spinach and carrot juice. Any other green veg-

preservatives, fillers, or coloring agents in processed foods. Be sure to read labels!

Acetaminophen	Food coloring
Aspirin	Formaldehyde
Baking powder	Ibuprofen
BHT (butylated hydroxytoluene)	MSG (monosodium glutamate)
Caffeine	Petroleum by-products
Drugs: over-the-counter,	Sodium benzoate
prescription, and street drugs	Tobacco

SIMPLE SUGGESTIONS FOR BREAKFAST AND SNACKS

People who are on Food Plan III and eat only Category I foods some-

etables can be used, such as green squash, collard greens, broccoli, and lettuce. Use just enough carrot juice to make it tasty, since carrot juice contains natural sugars, too much of which can be counterproductive.

A health food store carries green juices if you do not have a juicer. If the health food store does not carry green juices, sometimes they will order them for you. Read your label. You do not want fruit juice in this drink, just green juices and carrot juice.

Every day for three days drink: 1 quart or more of green juice with some carrot juice. Also drink 1 quart of distilled water or more. You may drink these juices any way you want. You can sip the juices all day or drink them every two hours. You can have the juices over ice, or dilute them with water. You can also have lemon water hot or cold.

After the green juice diet, I recommend that your first meal consist solely of steamed vegetables. For your second meal have raw vegetables, such as a salad. By your third meal, you can add some form of protein to your veggies, which can be cooked or raw.

By the second day of eating, you can eat all foods on Food Plan III. If you have a Body Chemistry test kit, start using it now to see if there are any foods on Food Plan III to which you react. For more on this, see page 212. You can start testing individual foods using the test kit and watching for symptoms.

times have difficulty with ideas for breakfast. Here are a few suggestions, many of which are also great as snacks.

❑ In the evening, cook some potatoes and refrigerate them. In the morning, slice them and sauté in butter.

❑ Baked potato with butter, guacamole, or pureed beans.

❑ Corn tortilla with butter, tomatoes, scrambled egg, and/or guacamole.

❑ Oatmeal with butter.

❑ Cream of Rice with butter.

❑ Rice cakes with sliced avocado, tomato, onion, green pepper, or cucumber.

❑ One-egg omelet with sliced tomato and diced vegetables (potato, green pepper, and onion are good choices).

❑ One-egg ranchero with corn tortilla.

❑ Cooked rice with butter.

❑ Steamed sweet potato with butter. (Sweet potatoes are also good cold. They taste like candy.)

❑ One cup of popped corn.

❑ Leftover rice heated with grated carrots, frozen peas, frozen lima beans, and butter. (This is my personal favorite.)

❑ Remember to always eat a starch with butter. The fat will help to regulate blood sugar and the blood sugar will not become elevated out of the normal range.

HEALTH-PROMOTING EATING HABITS

The following general health-promoting eating habits are beneficial on any food plan.

❑ Chew each mouthful of food at least twenty times.

❑ Do not wash foods down with liquids. Swallow your food before taking a drink.

❑ Consume portions that are easily digested.

❑ When emotionally upset or disturbed, eat smaller portions and chew food longer than usual.

❑ Do not overcook food.

❑ At each meal, consume as much raw food as cooked food.

❑ Rather than eating large meals less often, consume smaller meals more often.

❑ Examine each meal and snack from the following viewpoint: will any part of this meal upset my body chemistry?

❑ Eat small portions from a number of foods, rather than one large serving of a particular food.

Remove Sugar and Eat Whole Foods

Needless to say, I have a vendetta against sugar. It causes upset body chemistry that allows undigested food into the bloodstream. This causes inflammation in the bloodstream and all of its problems. Remove sugar from your diet. If you are still not convinced, read *Lick the Sugar Habit*. I have used much ink repeating this simple mantra: *Eat whole foods with limited or no processing.* Early man developed the ability to eat foods in certain chemical figurations, and modern food processing is a complete departure from this way of eating, changing the chemical configuration to weaken the effectiveness of digestive enzymes. Processed food can upset body chemistry, leading to toxicity, allergies, and difficulty in maintaining homeostasis. More prosaically, excessive effort to maintain homeostasis speeds up the body's aging process. Read and follow the food plans above for best results.

By following these good eating habits, you will lessen the incidence of body chemistry imbalance and facilitate more efficient digestion, assimilation, and utilization of nutrients. In addition, your body's ability to re-balance its chemistry in spite of other lifestyle insults will be supported. Response to appropriate medical care will be enhanced, as well. Now let's examine what you can do to further improve your lifestyle.

CREATING A HEALTHY LIFESTYLE

In addition to making a commitment to eat healthy, using the guidelines above, you must also commit to creating a lifestyle that promotes your well-being. The remainder of this chapter provides tips and suggestions for how you can most effectively do so. By implementing them, you will gain far greater control over your health.

Nutritional Supplements

Although many people have benefited from nutritional supplements, I am not in favor of using them at the expense of a healthy diet and lifestyle. Too often, supplements are used simply as an alternative to pharmaceutical pills, while the underlying dietary and lifestyle issues that need to be addressed are neglected. I do not approve of this approach to health. On the other hand, there is no question that different supplements can help, in certain cases, resolve certain deficiencies. Each person has different nutritional needs, however. These are best be determined by a health care practitioner trained in this area. Still, I do think it is a good idea to take a multivitamin and mineral supplement. For me this is like an insurance policy. Such products are available at your local health food store. Be sure you select one that is free of additives, fillers, and other items that you do not need, and to which your body may react. Avoid synthetic brands and choose food grade concentrates, instead, as these brands are better able to be utilized by our bodies. Read your label. There has been much research in medical journals on the two products that follow. I recommend both of them for inflammation.

Probiotics

Probiotics are microorganisms that contribute to the health and homeostasis of the internal flora, intestinal tract, and vagina. Referred to as friendly, beneficial, or good bacteria, the most frequently used probiotics are *lactobacilli* and *bifidobacteria.* Probiotics are usually used to protect a person from germs, and to improve the symptoms of irritable bowel syndrome, diarrhea, food allergy, eczema, *Candida albicans,* and lactose intolerance. They may also play a role in the management of gastric *Helicobacter pylori* infections, which are now recognized as the primary cause of ulcers. Certain research also suggests that probiotics may play a role in the prevention of carcinogenesis (cancer formation) and tumor growth.[1] Antibiotics kill off the good and bad bacteria, so always take probiotics with antibiotics to replenish your helpful bacteria. There are many brands that are made from a non-dairy base. Choose one of those.

Omega-3 Fatty Acids

Among the fatty acids, it is the omega-3 polyunsaturated fatty acids (PUFA) that possess the ability to help the immune system. Those from fish oil—eicosapentaenoic acid (EPA) and docosahexaenoic acid (DHA)—are the most biologically potent. Animal experiments and clinical intervention studies also indicate that omega-3 fatty acids have anti-inflammatory properties. Once you have found and stopped the cause of inflammation, omega-3 fatty acids can be beneficial in the healing process.

Coronary heart disease, major depression, aging, and cancer are all characterized by an increased level of interleukin, a proinflammatory cytokine. Similarly, arthritis, Crohn's disease, ulcerative colitis, and lupus are characterized by a high level of interleukin, as well as proinflammatory leukotrienes produced by omega-6 fatty acids. The primary sources of omega-6 are corn, soy, canola, safflower, and sunflower oil. These oils are overabundant in the diet and should be avoided or at least limited.

There have been a number of clinical trials assessing the benefits of adding fish oils to one's diet in order to combat several inflammatory diseases in humans, including rheumatoid arthritis, cancer, Crohn's disease, ulcerative colitis, psoriasis, lupus, multiple sclerosis, and migraine headaches. Many of the placebo-controlled trials of omega-3 in chronic inflammatory diseases reveal significant benefit, including decreased disease activity and a lowered use of anti-inflammatory drugs.[2]

Exercise

It has been known for a long time that when people exercise, the muscle cells use insulin more effectively, therefore delaying or preventing Type II diabetes from developing. Exercise may help control the inflammation process by reducing insulin resistance or improving vascular function, both factors that may help control the release of histamine and other substances that trigger an immune response. Exercise could also help control inflammation through a positive effect on body weight.

It has been stated that people with hypertension have increased inflammation. Exercise helps to bring down your blood pressure. At the American Academy of Sports Medicine, researchers found that exercising strenuously five to seven times a day lowered many people's blood pressure by 20 percent. In another study, a researcher from Tufts University found that participants who routinely engaged in vigorous exercise at least three days a week were about half as likely as others in the study to have elevated levels of C-reactive protein (CRP). However, more than 30 percent of the participants fell into the 'moderate activity' level—the steady walkers who worked out at least five times a week. These moderate exercisers showed greater benefit than light exercisers for levels of CRP.[3] The biggest problem is finding the exercise that fits your personality that you would want to do vigorously three to four times a week or more.

This research seems to show that, within reason, the more you exercise the less inflammation you have and the healthier you are. Three or more times a week, engage in some moderate to rigorous exercise for $1/2$ hour or more. I am sort of nuts on the subject. I climb 1,700 stairs, climb mountains, play tennis, and jog. I happen to like them all, but all you need is one that you like and will continue to do on a regular basis.

Those of you who do heavy-duty endurance exercises might put more stress on your body than is healthy. When a person over-exercises, not only can muscle damage occur, but also inflammation occurs through elevated cytokines.[4] If you regularly do marathons or other extreme exercise you might check with your health care practitioner about scheduling a CRP blood test (see Chapter 6).

Stop Smoking

Smoking causes the following: heart disease,[5] lung disease, systemic inflammation, nutritional abnormalities and weight loss, skeletal muscle dysfunction, and other problems.[6] Second hand smoking also has many implications, especially in children and young adults.[7] Stop smoking. With all the detrimental information concerning smoking, you must have a death wish to continue. There are many products now available to help you quit, as well as many websites and chatrooms you can visit for support. Many cities have programs that run in colleges, high schools, YMCAs, YWCAs, city parks, and other facilities to help smokers quit.

Read what even Philip Morris, the enemy, has to say about smoking and this might do it for you. "Philip Morris USA agrees with the overwhelming medical and scientific consensus that cigarette smoking causes lung cancer, heart disease, emphysema and other serious diseases in smokers. Smokers are far more likely to develop serious diseases, like lung cancer, than non-smokers. There is no safe cigarette."[8]

Reduce Alcohol Consumption

Studies of alcohol consumption can not seem to agree on one specific standard, some saying small amounts are good for the heart,[9] while others reject this. However, alcohol in a large quantity is uniformly frowned upon. As Dr. J. Davis wrote in his article, "Booze Could Be Tied to Allergy Blues," alcoholics have high levels of IgE antibodies in their blood, evidence of an extreme allergic response, inflammation, and a suppression of the immune system.[10] Alcohol seems to do its worst inflammatory damage when it kills bacteria living in the intestines, releasing endotoxins that tax the liver.[11]

I have been unable to find much research on other symptoms or diseases that might be the effect of excessive drinking of alcohol. It is necessary to research what the relationship is of drinking alcohol to cancer, diabetes, Alzheimer's disease, and other diseases than heart disease. Here are a few examples on which I can speak.

Beer and wine use sulfites during production. Many asthmatics and people with chemical sensitivities react to these sulfites.[12] Drinking alcohol can cause the nasal-sinus membranes to swell, trapping air and mucus, causing inflammation behind the narrowed openings of the sinuses. If the sinus openings become too narrow to permit drainage of the mucus, then bacteria begin to multiply. The bacteria didn't get you. You created this mess with alcohol.[13] *Candida albicans* can also become a problem when alcohol is consumed habitually over a lifetime. Probiotics can help this from happening but stopping excessive drinking is even a better solution.

For some people, an allergy to grapes, barley, or some other grain that is used in making alcohol could be a problem. If you have symptoms or an undisclosed problem resulting from a blood test, you might remove alcohol from your diet for a week. After you do so, see if your blood test returns to homeostasis and/or your symptoms go away. If so, this is a sure sign that you should eliminate alcohol from your lifestyle.

Reduce Stress

We have established that distress causes the inflammatory process. Distress also reduces hormones that stop inflammation. Findings show psychological stress can influence the onset and/or progression of conditions that involve excessive inflammation, such as allergic, autoimmune, cardiovascular, infections, and rheumatoid illnesses.[14]

The good news is that social support lessens the consequences of stress, perhaps by helping people better deal with economic, work, and family disruptions that cause stress in the first place.[15] We all need support from family and friends. Make sure you stay in contact with your family and find and join groups that share your interests and activities. Love and support help to alleviate the pain of stress. Here are other simple steps you can take to better manage stress:

- Eat a healthy diet (see Food Plans).

- Do exercises that you enjoy, and that are appropriate for your age and current health condition. Exercising regularly is an excellent way to relieve stress.

- Cultivate interests, hobbies, and diversions outside of your work, and engage in them regularly.

- Get enough sleep (see below).

- Laugh. Laughter is an excellent way of releasing tension.

- Consider learning stress-reduction techniques, such as meditation, biofeedback, breathing techniques, yoga, or Tai chi.

Sleep Well and Enough

Sleep plays an important role in homeostasis, so do not deny yourself sleep for extended periods of time. A preliminary study of eleven healthy young men who underwent sleep deprivation (four hours/day) for six nights followed by sleep recovery (twelve hours/day) for seven nights found significant metabolic and hormonal changes. Glucose or blood sugar metabolism during the sleep-deprived state resembled that typical in unhealthy adults and those with Type II diabetes. Those people who are deprived of sleep for long periods of time can have a decreased thyroid hormone, fluxuations in corticosteroids, high blood pressure, and memory difficulties.[16]

Melatonin is a powerful hormone that has helped some people with sleep problems. I do not recommend it, but if you take it for any period of time your blood level for melatonin should be checked. You might try L-tryptophan, an amino acid and melatonin precursor that might also help build up your melatonin levels.

Dr. Joseph Mercola, author of *The No-Grain Diet* and publisher of the website www.mercola.com, recommends these additional tips for ensuring a restful, good night's sleep:

1. Sleep in complete darkness.

2. Avoid watching television before bedtime or reading stimulating books, as both can cause stimulating effects on the brain and interfere with your sleep cycle.

3. If you suffer from cold feet, wear socks to bed.

4. Regularly participate in spiritual or religious activities (reading scriptures, praying, meditating, expressing gratitude), which can help you surrender to a blessing of well-earned rest.

5. Don't use loud alarm clocks. Waking up suddenly is stressful. If you regularly get enough sleep, your body will learn to awaken naturally.

6. Go to bed early to allow your body systems, including the adrenals, gallbladder, and liver, to dump toxins and recharge, which they most effectively do between 11 P.M. and 1 A.M. If you're awake during this time, the toxins back up into your entire system, disrupting your health.

7. Keep your bedroom temperature at 70 degrees or less.

8. Reduce or avoid the use of prescription and over-the-counter medications, as these can affect sleep.

9. Avoid caffeine.

10. Keep electrical devices at least three feet from the bed to allow your body complete rest. (This includes your electric blanket. If you want a warm bed before you get in, turn on the electric blanket but turn it off and unplug it before your get in.)

11. Avoid drinking two hours before bedtime to reduce your need to go to the bathroom during sleep time.

12. Take a hot bath, shower, or sauna before retiring. This temporary rise in body temperature facilitates sleep.

13. Make your bedroom solely a place for sleeping. If you watch TV or work in bed, you'll find it harder to associate your bedroom as a place to relax and sleep.

14. If you're menopausal or perimenopausal, get checked out by a good natural medicine physician, since hormonal changes at this time may cause insomnia if not properly addressed.[17]

Regain and Maintain Your Optimal Weight

Obesity plays a giant role in the degenerative disease process. Most obese people have inflammation, are more allergic to foods, have AGEs, and show vulnerability to free radicals, so it would seem prudent to maintain your optimal weight. One research paper showed that when overweight people were given 4 grams of fish oils per day, there was no difference in their CRP levels.[18] If you continue to eat junk food and stay overweight, taking fish oil pills will not work, nor will anything else. First things first, lose weight. Food Plan III above (see page 133) works wonders for weight loss. It fills you up, but not out. If you get hungry between meals, just eat another meal from Food Plan III. Also follow my suggestions for breakfasts and snacks beginning on page 138.

Health is definitely a holistic approach that is best achieved when we make a personal commitment to being healthy. If you are presently unhealthy, you need to shape up in all areas or you might ship out earlier than you would like, with leaky broken parts as well. Fortunately, you can avoid this by following all of the above guidelines.

8

Detoxification
for Health

Removing toxins from the body is an important step in healing. I have asked an authority to write about detoxification and how it can keep inflammation under control. The following is written by Carolyn Dean MD, ND, an expert in this area.

OUR TOXIC WORLD

The word *detoxification* is derived from the Latin *toxicum* or poison; it means to deprive of poisonous qualities. The Oxford English Dictionary (OED) puts *detoxicate* in common usage from 1867. Throughout the next few decades, according to the OED, *detoxification* was used to describe the body's ability to neutralize various drugs and chemicals, such as pesticides. But by the 1970s, detoxification became mostly associated with drug and alcohol rehabilitation, and that is the inference people now make when they hear the word. But detoxification is not just an externally imposed therapeutic method offered at a local detoxification clinic. Detoxification is performed every minute of every day by our various organs in an orchestration worthy of Carnegie Hall.

Inflammation has been well defined in this book. Detoxification can be described as the process of preventing inflammation. As has been stated, although inflammation may come across as the bad guy with its redness, heat, swelling, and pain, we can not forget that inflammation is trying to help us by localizing and eradicating the "foreign" substance and repairing the surrounding damaged tissue. Inflammation is a necessary and beneficial process, but if we keep immersing ourselves in various toxins that cause inflammation, then the inflammatory process is going to get out of control.

We have good reason to worry about toxins and to be concerned about our body's ability to detoxify them. The role of the U.S. Environmental Protection Agency (EPA) should be to stem the tide of chemicals that overflow into our world, but it seems that they do little more than count the flowing barrels of pollutants. According to 2000 EPA statistics, more than 4 billion pounds of chemicals were released into the earth that year, contaminating ground water, and seeping into wells and reservoirs. Another 250 million pounds of chemicals were "legally" discharged into surface waters (e.g. lakes and rivers) by industry and around dumpsites. And 2 billion pounds of air emissions were pumped into the atmosphere. Add to that the thousands of pounds of food additives that are deliberately added to our food supply, and another few thousand that make their way in as trace amounts of herbicides, pesticides, and food-processing chemicals. Four hundred licensed pesticides amount to 2.5 billion pounds each year, choking the life out of any land still able to grow living plants. Helping to sweeten the fourteen pounds of food additives, the average American eats 154 pounds of sugar every year.

Our environment, according to science and medicine, is something that we should control; it should not control us. I am afraid both science and medicine are sadly mistaken. From industrial effluent polluting rivers and oceans and making fish unsafe to eat; to industrial smoke stacks polluting the air and giving us acid rain and acid soil; to the more than 50,000 chemicals in daily use; to food additives; thousands of prescription and over-the-counter drugs; artificial sweeteners; aluminum cooking utensils; household chemicals; pesticides and herbicides; and mercury deliberately put in our dental fillings, vaccines, and medicines—we are living in a toxic nation and a toxic planet.

As reported by noted Canadian activist and medical journalist, Helke Ferrie, "Our bodies have become the world's toxic dump sites. The billions of dollars worth of pesticides, plastics, petroleum products, and heavy-metal containing technology have made the industrial world rich beyond belief, and threaten human survival as it conquers the earth. As in the story of King Midas, whose touch turned everything to gold—even his wife and children—our economy is killing us." Dr. Sherry Rogers in her recent publication, *Detoxify or Die,* pulls no punches. She says, "We have conquered the world with pollution. There are no more pristine areas left without a trace of man's manufacturing might."

Dr. Samuel Epstein, Professor of Environmental and Occupational Medicine, University of Illinois School of Public Health, led the fight to remove DDT from America, although it is still used in other countries. Dr. Epstein maintains that each one of us harbors 500 different chemicals in all the cells of our body. The Environmental Protection Agency confirms that 100 percent of the world's population harbors traces of heavy metals like mercury, lead, and cadmium in their blood. Dr. Rogers echoes this warning and writes that, "Indeed every living thing now has DDT in its tissues and its toxic effects are increasing over time." Helke Ferrie reports that the World Health Organization admits that, in terms of scientific research on environment pollution, there are no more "control groups" free of toxic synthetic chemicals to be found in the world.

Brain, bowel, and hormonal organs, including testicles and ovaries, are all equally affected. Our body ineffectually lashes out against the invasion of chemicals that it was never equipped to handle. The result is inflammation followed by epidemics of allergies, arthritis, autoimmune disease, cancer, chronic fatigue syndrome, mood disorders, and neurological diseases that, as Helke Ferrie says, "no amount of fancy genetics will explain away."[1]

Environmental illness is barely recognized by the medical community, however. The trend of the past decade is to put illnesses caused by environmental factors into a category of "autoimmune disease." Neurosurgeon Russell Blaylock, in a 2002 lecture, reminds us that we are not immune to ourselves if we have a healthy body but we do set up an immune reaction to an "abnormal self" riddled with inflammation, toxins, and antigen/antibody reactions to these toxins and inflammatory products.

All body tissues are subject to damage by free radicals. A free radical is an unstable molecule that has an unpaired electron that steals a stabilizing electron from another molecule potentially causing cell damage. External sources of free radicals are what we now identify as environmental pollutants. The usual way to study chemical pollution has been to measure our water and air, and to determine the levels that might cause harm. There are few studies that measure the people that are bathing and breathing in pollutants.

Merely setting "so-called" safe limits has not prevented the chemicals themselves from entering our bodies.

A certain percentage of people take measures to counteract the toxins and poisons, but even they can not help but trap chemicals in their system. In a 2003 landmark study led by New York's Mount Sinai School of Medicine, in collaboration with the Environmental Working Group (EWG) and Commonweal, researchers at two major laboratories measured the levels of chemicals in a group of human beings. The researchers found "an average of 91 industrial compounds, pollutants, and other chemicals in the blood and urine of nine volunteers, with a total of 167 chemicals found in the group. Like most of us, the people tested do not work with chemicals on the job and do not live near an industrial facility."

The EWG said that scientists characterize this contamination as a person's "body burden." They further cautioned, "Of the 167 chemicals found, 76 cause cancer in humans or animals, 94 are toxic to the brain and nervous system, and 79 cause birth defects or abnormal development. The dangers of exposure to these chemicals in combination has never been studied."

HOW TOXINS BUILD UP IN OUR BODIES

We only have to follow the scenario of a human life on our planet to enumerate the ways toxins build up in our body. A newborn infant, Annie, is injected with several vaccines (preserved with mercury) before leaving the hospital. Her mother drinks diet soda (containing the neurotoxin, aspartame, which is created from two brain stimulating amino acids and wood alcohol) and eats food loaded with additives (such as the excitotoxin MSG) that pass into her breast milk and into her child's fragile brain and liver. Actually, Annie is already saturated with the toxins that her mother ate while she was pregnant. One of the worst is mercury found in the tuna fish sandwiches that her mother eats almost every day. Annie's immune system is weakened by the vaccinations (besides mercury, they contain aluminum and several other chemicals).

Due to her weakened immune system, Annie develops an ear infection when she is only one month old; for this she is put on antibiotics. Because the antibiotic kills off all the normal bacteria in her intestines she develops an overgrowth of *Candida* yeast and gets diarrhea and a diaper rash. Medicine for the diarrhea and a cortisone ointment for the rash do not help very much, but increase Annie's toxic load. Consequently, she develops eczema, which is really from *Candida* toxins (see page 68), and is put on more cortisone creams, which feed the yeast. It is no coincidence that suppressing the eczema had turned into asthma. Annie also seems to become more hyperactive after eating sugar, and gets diarrhea when she eats too much bread, and constipation after too much dairy.

All this goes unnoticed by her parents and her doctor. The ear infections and the antibiotics continue until her doctor decides to put tubes in Annie's ears. The anesthetic during surgery has to be detoxified in the liver and Annie's asthma gets worse. She is on several inhalers and has spent many nights in the emergency ward.

When Annie enters preschool, she is exposed to germs from her classmates and comes down with more colds and flu. She develops a host of allergies including unrecognized food allergies. By her teens Annie is pale and looks undernourished but overweight. Her favorite foods are pizza, hamburgers, and anything with sugar. She develops cold sores on her lips and gets several attacks a year. She eats no vegetables, little fruit, and drinks too much soda. She alternates between regular soda with 8–10 teaspoons of sugar, or diet soda with aspartame. Her health and her teeth suffer; Annie has ten mercury amalgam fillings by the age of 14. She becomes even more apathetic and seems tired all the time and sleeps about fourteen hours a day. When her period comes, it is a disaster. She has cramps and irregular bleeding and yeast infections. Her doctor suggests the birth control pill to help stop the pain and "regulate" her periods. In her first year in college Annie contracts mononucleosis and lies in bed for six months. She still has allergies, asthma, frequent infections, and now is chronically fatigued.

Annie does not go back to college, but takes a beautician's course that exposes her daily to toxic chemicals from nail polish, nail glue, nail polish removers, hair dyes, and hair processing chemicals. When she gets married, Annie finds that her chronic yeast infections from taking antibiotics four or more times a year makes sexual intercourse very painful. And she is unable to get pregnant. Perhaps because she took the Pill before her own menstrual cycle developed, she does not ovulate. Now Annie has to take fertility drugs in order for her to conceive, but the drugs make her nauseous and even more miserable, with swollen breasts and fluid retention. Her one and only pregnancy is very difficult. She develops eclampsia with high blood pressure, painful edema and gains fifty pounds.

Annie is never able to lose the weight and by age 40 she is diabetic, and has ulcerative colitis, fibrositis, and chronic fatigue. She drinks coffee to keep herself awake through the day, eats mostly bread and pasta, liters of diet soda a day, and has strong sugar cravings. She convinces herself she is trying to be healthy by eating mostly "diet" food products laced with the synthetic sweetener, aspartame. She does not realize that aspartame is causing her to have daily headaches, muscle aches and pains, and actually causes more sugar cravings. For her pain she takes the maximum daily dose of several painkillers. And, in spite of her allergies, Annie smokes, because she says it helps deal with the constipation that is part of her ulcerative colitis picture.

Unfortunately, we all know people who fit this horrific profile. It may even fit you. Annie had all the common symptoms of toxic build-up, including fatigue, muscle aches and pains, repeated colds, joint pain, allergy symptoms, insomnia, back pain, mood swings, arthritis symptoms, constipation, sinus congestion, and headaches. Each ache and pain is a point of inflammation in the body from the build-up of toxins and the inability of Annie's body to clear them.

Her immune system is also toxic and has been from an early age, leaving her with symptoms of asthma, allergies, eczema, and chronic infections. Fat-soluble toxins such as organophosphate pesticides and the "excitotoxins" MSG and aspartame gravitate to the brain, leading to neurological toxicity affecting mood, memory and behavior. Yeast by-products include the very toxic acetaldehyde and other chemicals that mimic hormones, causing hormonal dysfunction. Annie's hormonal symptoms include PMS, dysmenorrhea, infertility, and lack of sex drive. After decades of sugar addiction and a fifty pound weight gain, it is no wonder that Annie develops insulin resistance and diabetes.

Yet, allopathic medicine, in its unwavering focus on treating the symptoms of disease with suppressive drugs, pays no attention to the common scenario that Annie and thousands of her peers are experiencing. Medicine also pays little attention to the body's detoxification systems. It is not a specific topic in medical school; there are no specific allopathic tests for toxicity; and there are no "drugs" to treat toxic overload. In fact, drugs, whether prescription or over-the-counter, must all be detoxified in the liver, placing more stress on a system already burdened with the overabundance of chemicals in our environment.

HOW THE BODY DETOXIFIES

Any foreign material that gains access to our body can cause inflammation and must necessarily be dealt with by our immune system and our detoxification system. But we need to be aware of how our organs of detoxification perform the miracle of cleansing our body so we can understand how to support this process. In general, the body is able to detoxify the basic end products of daily metabolism. Most of the biochemical pathways have mechanisms that reconstitute enzymes, and vitamin and mineral co-factors that are used in the process, like a self-perpetuating system. All sense of that is lost when the body also has to detoxify large amounts of external chemicals. Once the enzymes and vitamin and mineral co-factors are used up and flushed out, and not replaced, this leads to eventual depletion.

The actual process of detoxification in the liver is fascinating. It basically entails the conversion of fat-soluble toxins into water-soluble metabolites, which are usually, but not always, less toxic. Water-soluble chemicals can then be excreted through the kidneys, whereas fat-soluble chemicals cannot. If they are not converted they are either dumped into the intestines with the bile or end up being stored in fatty tissue. Many people who understand the process of toxicity in the body feel that the epidemic of obesity is, in part, due to the body's need for a place to store the chemicals to which it is exposed. For that reason, if you are overweight, and trying to detoxify, you have to proceed cautiously so that you are not overwhelmed by all of the toxins being liberated from shrinking fat cells. The feeling of being poisoned causes many people to abandon their goal of losing weight.

Detoxification occurs mostly in the liver, with some activity in the blood, lungs, and walls of the intestine. In the liver it is talked about as phases. Phase I occurs in the liver cell membrane. Dozens of different enzymes act on chemicals, adding or taking away an oxygen or hydrogen molecule to make the chemical water-soluble. This phase of activity depends on co-factors in the form of vitamins, minerals, amino acids, and hormones. Detoxification can be seriously hampered if there are deficiencies. The B vitamins, vitamin C, and progesterone are the most important co-factors involved in the process of converting fat-soluble toxins to water-soluble ones. Underactive or overactive Phase I function can be a problem. Poor Phase I functioning creates an inability to tolerate caffeine, while overactive Phase I means you can have a high tolerance for caffeine. Underactive Phase I means you just are not detoxifying chemicals and the overload can damage the liver and lead to autoimmune disease. If Phase I is overactive, you detoxify chemicals too rapidly and end up with an excess of very unstable chemicals waiting to be further processed through the Phase II pathway. If Phase II is under-functioning, when you eat asparagus you get strong smelling urine and you may be sensitive to sulfites.

Phase II detoxification is slightly more complicated, with certain molecules attaching to the Phase I products making them more water-soluble and easier to eliminate. This phase depends on sulphur obtained from the diet. Cruciferous vegetables, such as broccoli, cabbage, and Brussels sprouts, are sulphur-containing foods and have been widely promoted as immune-boosting and health-promoting. That is because they help the liver in its ability to detoxify.

Many toxins, such as petrochemical hydrocarbons, pharmaceutical drugs, and steroid hormones, do not allow molecules to be added or taken away and do not allow themselves to be turned into a water-soluble waste product. Those chemicals require sulfur amino acids (amino acids are the building blocks of protein) that grab onto these toxic chemicals and convey a "stickiness" that drags them out of the body when the sulphur amino acid is excreted. Sulphur amino acids like methionine, cysteine, and n-acetyl-cysteine (NAC) are so powerful that they can pull out mercury, lead, and arsenic. Conjugation with glutathione, an important body detoxifier, requires vitamins B_6 and B_{12}, folate, and magnesium.

You can see the delicate orchestration required to cleanse the body and maintain homeostasis. Detoxification can not proceed normally when the Phase I and II pathways are overloaded with external chemicals and heavy metals, or when the body does not receive the necessary vitamins and minerals in the diet. It is only when we agree that toxins are building up in our bodies and are a potential problem that we can turn our attention to trying to get rid of them through detoxification.

HELPING THE BODY TO DETOXIFY

The major focus of detoxification is to:

1. Identify the toxins and decrease the exposure.

2. Maximize excretion of the toxin.

3. Provide nutritional support for specific detoxification pathways.

4. Re-establish intestinal flora balance.

Exposure to toxins can come from air, food, and water. To identify the culprit, in the larger sense, you must find out what industry or business is behind the contamination. It will not suffice to just try and clean your own personal environment and body; that would be an endless task. We have to treat the cause and actively work to try to eliminate chemicals in our environment.

Personal cleansing should begin with decreasing food toxins. Food Plan III (see Chapter 6) is an effective detoxification diet. Many people will go through withdrawal symptoms by going on this diet. The reason for this is that you are removing junk foods and many empty-calorie foods from your diet. It has been scientifically shown that with a whole food diet and getting off the junk, you can dramatically slow down aging and disease. This translates into a small miracle—nothing that any medicine or gene therapy is capable of even coming close to duplicating.

To take the above diet one step further and to ensure that we are not eating foods that are high in pesticides and herbicides means going organic and making meals from scratch. Going organic and eating wholesome food does not mean you have to become a vegetarian. You need high-biological-value protein to create the necessary detoxification molecules in the liver and people in the "O" group (according to The Blood Group Diet theory of Drs. James and Peter D'Adamo) need animal protein. Between 70 and 75 percent of the population is "O" type blood group.[2]

Other steps in the detoxification process include maximizing excretion of the toxin through specific detoxification procedures. These include dry saunas, infrared saunas, steam baths, bathing, sweating, exercise, colonics, enemas, and chelation therapy. Herbal remedies taken both orally and via herbal pads applied to the feet to draw out toxins can also be employed.

Dry Saunas

Although called a dry sauna, presumably to differentiate from steam baths, it is important to have some humidity in the sauna because extreme dryness can irritate the lungs. Saunas make you sweat and sweat supposedly carries toxins out of the body. Most health clubs and spas have saunas rooms or you can install a small sauna in your own home. Take a shower first and sit on a towel on one of the wooden benches. The upper bench will be hotter since heat rises. As your skin temperature elevates your pores open and sweat will trickle down your body. The usual temperature of a sauna is between 120–150 degrees Fahrenheit. A slightly higher temperature can be reached by throwing water on the heating stones to create steam and humidity.

Some people claim that the slight elevation of body temperature by one to three degrees sufficiently mimics a fever. It is well known to naturopaths that a fever is one defense against viral and bacterial infection. The heat itself is relaxing for tired and achy muscles and is beneficial for stress reduction.

After five or ten minutes you can cool down with a shower and come back into the sauna for another few minutes. This cycle can be repeated several times. Drink plenty of water after a sauna to replace what you lose from sweating. Short saunas are beneficial to most people. However, there are special sauna programs using lower temperatures but longer times, under a doctor's supervision, for drug, chemical, and heavy metal detoxification. Presently over one hundred firemen in New York are undergoing sauna therapy as part of their detoxification program after being sickened in the 9/11 cleanup.

Because heat dilates blood vessels, people with low blood pressure should be very careful to take very short saunas. A headache or a feeling of faintness may indicate that the blood pressure is falling. Similarly, if you have not eaten before your sauna, increased metabolism caused by the heat can drop your blood sugar.

Far Infrared Saunas

The same principles of heat dilating the blood vessels and causing sweating apply to the infrared sauna. However, the heating source, instead of being the traditional wood and stones or the more modern electrically heated stones, is known as far infrared technology. Far infrared saunas work by heating the body, while the surrounding air remains relatively cool. Sweating begins quickly and without the discomfort of intense heat. Far infrared saunas are becoming very popular and I predict that the industry will be able to support research studies to show the benefits of far infrared sauna therapy for detoxification.

Steam Baths

Steam baths use wet heat and are the modern day version of Native American sweat lodges. The lodges served as ritual cleansing but also cleansed the skin and created a significant amount of sweating, and presumably toxin release, in the process. Many health professional recommend steam baths today for this same reason.

Bathing

If you do not have access to a sauna or a steam bath you can still create your own spa in your bathroom. It is preferable if you have a filter on your shower and fill your tub that way to avoid bathing in chlorinated water. Add Epsom salts to your bath. I use about two cups in my baths but you might want to start with $1/4$ cup. Epson salts are magnesium sulfate and are absorbed to a certain extent. In my book, *The Miracle of Magnesium*, I write about a case of a woman who used so much Epsom salts in a bath that she got loose bowel movements! Magnesium sulfate is a strong laxative as well as being a powerful muscle relaxant. You can also add aromatherapy oils to your bath for relaxation or for energy. Water from boiling several slices of ginger confers more healing and detoxification benefits to your bath.

Exercise

If it makes you sweat then it is going to help you. And when you exercise, deep breathing is not far behind! It is little known that the lymphatic system, which drains away cellular metabolic wastes, is actively massaged by deep breathing. Shallow breathing moves some air in and out of only a portion of the lungs, but deep breathing can oxygenate twice as much blood by expanding the lungs fully. This fully renewed and revitalized blood brings greater nourishment to every cell in the body.

Colonics

Some of the old time herbalists remind us that "death begins in the colon." This may seem a bit extreme, but remember, in the large intestine, fecal matter is compacted and fluids are reabsorbed into the body so the stools will not be watery. If those intestinal fluids are composed of toxic materials, some of them will be reabsorbed into the bloodstream. Simply think of a heavy meal of meat, bread and fat that first creates heartburn and inflammation, then gas, then constipation as it heaves its way to the large intestine. Incompletely digested food is preyed upon by yeasts and bacteria in the intestines, making chemical by-products with descriptive names such as putrescine and cadaverine—described as having the smell of rotting flesh! The longer these chemicals stay in the intestines the more opportunity there is for them to be reabsorbed into the body.

High colonic enemas, administered by a nurse or a trained colon therapist, is a form of intestinal detoxification. When my grandmother was a nurse in a "fever hospital" high colonic enemas were considered a normal hospital procedure. They were also routinely used before abdominal surgery to ensure a clean bowel.

Such an enema is given while lying comfortably on an examining table. A nozzle connected to a long tube and heated filtered water is lubricated and inserted into the anus. You may be asked to lie on your left side and then on your back as water fills up the large intestine. At any point when slight pressure builds up, the water is allowed to flow back out. Over a period of about forty-five minutes the entire large intestine is cleaned. During a detoxification protocol one or more colonic enemas can be helpful to enhance the process. Make sure you go to a trained colon therapist who used filtered water and disposable nozzles.

Enemas

Saline enemas, bought in pharmacies, and coffee enemas, prepared at home, are usually self-administered. Coffee enemas are recommended by doctors, most notably Dr. Nicholas Gonzalez, for detoxification for patients undergoing cancer therapy. The caffeine, theophylline, and theobromines contained in coffee are absorbed by the large collection of veins near the anus and cause smooth muscle relaxation in blood vessels and the bile duct. This stimulates the expulsion of bile from the liver and gall bladder.

You can buy a reusable enema bag in a pharmacy. It resembles a hot water bottle with a hose at the end. The recipe for the enema uses filtered water and organic coffee. Boil 4 cups of water and add 3 tablespoons of coffee. Boil for three minutes and simmer for twenty. Strain and cool to body temperature.

Make yourself comfortable on blankets and a towel on the floor. Learn how to adjust the shut off valve, lubricate the nozzle, and insert into the anus. Lie on your left side and release the valve. Close the valve if you feel pressure and lie on your back and open the valve again. Then move to your right side. Try to retain the coffee for ten to fifteen minutes. A coffee enema is best done after you have had your normal morning bowel movement and should not interfere with your bowel movement the next morning.

Chelation Therapy

Intravenous chelation therapy is a medical treatment performed in a doctor's office that can improve metabolic function and blood flow through blocked arteries in the body by pulling out heavy metals. In my book, *The Everything Alzheimer's Book,* I reported a recent study from the December 2003 issue of *Archives of Neurology* on chelation.

Using a drug called clioquinol, researchers found that it lowered levels of amyloid in people with moderately severe forms of Alzheimer's and improved their mental function tests.

Researchers who think the underlying cause of Alzheimer's is the build-up of beta-amyloid protein feel this chelation study proves their theory that, by chelating out the protein, there is improvement in mental function. However Dr. Boyd Haley, of the University of Kentucky, takes the other side of the argument. He is convinced that, since chelation treatment pulls out heavy metals, it may work by preventing zinc and copper from binding to amyloid, thereby dissolving it and preventing build-up. Dr. Haley reminds us that it is copper, zinc, and mercury that are present in dental fillings and present in amyloid plaque that are being chelated out of the brain and causing the improvement in mental function. Dr. Haley's research shows that mercury damage to brain nerve cells is exactly the same damage as seen in Alzheimer's brains on autopsy.

On a more personal note, Tom Warren became his own expert in such things as chelation and dental fillings after being diagnosed with Alzheimer's. As part of his investigations he had a CT scan that showed brain atrophy consistent with Alzheimer's. Mr. Warren did a lot of investigations of his own and tried a number of therapies, including chelation therapy and having his mercury dental fillings removed. After four years he was symptom-free and his CT scan was normal. He wrote *Beating Alzheimer's: A Step Towards Unlocking the Mysteries of Brain Diseases* to help other people find their way to better health.

Presently there are several drugs that are used as chelators. In fact, clioquinol, used in the 2003 study, may not be the most powerful or beneficial. Ethylene-diamine-tetra-acetic acid (EDTA), Dimercaptosuccinic Acid (DMSA), and Sodium Dimercaptopropanesulfonate (DMPS) are the three most commonly used chelating agents for heavy metals.

Because of the invasive nature of intravenous chelation and the use of chelating drugs that may have side effects, protocols using natural chelating substances are being researched. The following are some of the recommendations for carrying out an "oral chelation" program.

- Make sure you have sufficient protein and plants with sulfur amino acids: eggs, broccoli, Brussels sprouts, cabbage. Fasting during detoxification means you will not have sufficient sulfur molecules to neutralize the toxins that are being released from fat cells and other storage sites.

- Using fiber and enemas, make sure you are having several bowel movements a day to hasten the elimination of toxins.

- Take a multi-vitamin/mineral, preferably one that is food-based.

- Use mercury detox agents such as: cilantro, garlic, and onions.

- Use milk thistle herb for liver support during detoxification.

- Glutathione is one of the most powerful antioxidants in the body. It is mostly available as an intravenous treatment but is being studied in its sublingual form.

Probiotics and Prebiotics

In many instances, the body will just begin its healing journey through Food Plan III and a green juice fast. Besides the recommendations for oral chelation it is important to re-establish intestinal flora balance by introducing natural probiotics. (Also see Chapter 7.) Probiotics is the name given to intestinal bacteria that have a beneficial role in the body. Most people who are aware of probiotics know them as acidophilus that is found in yogurt. There are dozens of other beneficial bacteria and a huge scientific inquiry is elucidating their value.

A recent paper in a 2004 gastroenterology journal article on probiotics and prebiotics in gastrointestinal disorders shows that the medical establishment is actively involved in this research.[3] Prebiotics are foods or nutrients that are used by specific bacteria and that can be added to the diet to increase the chances of these particular bacteria growing and thriving in the intestine. Fructooligosaccharides (FOS) is one of the prebiotics. The paper is actually a review that summarizes the clinical effects of probiotics and prebiotics in gastrointestinal disorders and describes how they work.

For decades it was thought that probiotics simply worked to protect the gut by acting as a barrier to harmful bacteria. However, research now shows that probiotic bacteria modulate mucosal and systemic immune activity and epithelial function. The reviewers reported that enough "evidence now exists for the therapeutic use of probiotics in infectious diarrhea in children, recurrent *Clostridium difficile*-induced infections and postoperative pouchitis." They also revealed that "evidence is emerging for the use of probiotics in other gastrointestinal infections, prevention of postoperative bacterial translocation, irritable bowel syndrome, and in both ulcerative colitis and Crohn disease."

AVOIDING TOXINS—THE DOS AND DON'TS

The following are some potentially damaging practices to avoid and action steps you can take to minimize your exposure to toxins and prevent disease.[4]

- Do not smoke, or tolerate smoking in your family's presence.

- Avoid excessive exposure to sunlight and ultraviolet rays.

- Do not consider breast implants.

- Do not use dark hair dyes; check out safe alternatives.

- Avoid perfumes, air-fresheners, and perfumed deodorizers and antiperspirants. If they contain benzene, aluminum, lemon-scented chemicals, or lack a full list of all ingredients to permit a check-up in a toxicology manual—do not use them.

- Treat all cosmetic products with extreme suspicion until you have proof positive that they contain no known carcinogens; safe alternatives exist.

- Avoid dry-cleaned clothes, look for non-chemical alternatives.

- Avoid chlorinated water.

- Do not drink fluoridated water or use fluoridated toothpaste.

- Avoid electromagnetic fields (EMUs), especially with children. EMUs have been linked to childhood leukemia and brain cancers. Use appropriate protection on your computer screen, avoid using a microwave oven, and avoid living near hydro towers.

- Do not use hormone disrupting or mimicking substances such as chemical pesticides, herbicides, fertilizers, fungicides and bug killers.

- Do not use cleaning, polishing, renovation materials in your home that list unspecified "inert ingredients." If they have toxic warning symbols; require calling a doctor; are "corrosive"; give special disposal instructions; or require "well-ventilated areas" for use—look for substitutes. If you cannot avoid some of these substances (e.g. oil paint, furniture stripper, car maintenance materials, etc.), wear the best charcoal-filtered mask available and minimize exposure, especially to skin and lungs.

- Reduce consumption of salt-cured, smoked, and nitrate-cured foods.

- Do not use the meat from animals routinely treated with antibiotics and raised with hormones. Meat from range-fed animals are widely available in health food stores and some grocery stores.

- Never heat shrink-wrapped foods or food in plastic containers. The plastic molecules migrate into the food when heated.

- Avoid food additives, especially Red Dye No. 3 found in most junk foods and many pop products. Avoid emulsifiers such as carrageenin; do not consume hydrogenated vegetable oils or margarine.

- Limit sport fish consumption to the guidelines provided seasonally by the government.

- Do not drink or eat foods that contain sugar substitutes such as NutraSweet, Aspartame, and Sucralose. Stevia is a healthy substitute.

- Avoid antibiotics unless your doctor has done the necessary test to identify the exact bacteria this antibiotic kills (except in extreme emergencies, e.g. meningitis); keep treatment period to a minimum.

- Avoid prescription drugs unless your doctor also gives you a copy of the full drug information from the annually updated PDR (Physicians Desk Reference) and explains this information to you; if the drug requires regular liver function tests, insist on discussing alternatives or keep treatment to the minimum.

- Avoid birth control pills, antihypertensives, antidepressants, hormone replacement therapy in pill form (toxic to the liver), and do not take Tamoxifen preventively; get the full data on those drugs; check them out first on the Internet at www.preventcancer.com.

- Do not invest in companies and industry sectors that are known cancer source polluters.

Do Something Constructive About Toxins You Already Have

1. Have your mercury amalgams removed by a dentist trained in the proper protocol.

2. If you are overweight, have your hormone levels checked and find out if you have food allergies; over-exposure to estrogen; lack of progesterone; thyroid problems brought on by pesticide exposure; or an adaptation to allergenic foods (often wheat products and refined sugar are frequent cause of obesity, which promote cancer through excessive estrogen and pesticide storage).

3. Exercise regularly and moderately.

4. Eat cruciferous vegetables (cauliflower, Brussels sprouts, broccoli, etc.) preferably from organically grown sources; if that doesn't fit your budget, wash all your fruits and vegetables in VegiWash. This will remove pesticide surface residues.

5. Buy your foods in glass containers, avoid cans and plastic.

6. Join a health or cancer activist group.

7. Start a pesticide education group in your neighborhood, demand from your local representatives mandatory toxicology disclosure of all chemical ingredients being sold today; approach your local golf course manager and discuss alternative ways of maintenance; go to your city council and get them to explore alternatives to chlorine in public swimming pools and to put a stop to the use of chlorine and fluoride in the water supply.

8. Don't go shopping without *Dr. Epstein's Safe Shoppers Bible,* 2nd ed. 1999, or *Additive Alert,* Alive publications, 1999.

According to Dr. Epstein, other toxic substances and activities you can choose to avoid include all contraceptives, hormones, HRT; food additives, aspartame, and food dyes; fluorides; premenopausal mammography; silicon implants; animal fats derived from animals fed hormones and antibiotics; estrogenic pesticides; bovine growth hormones injected into commercially raised dairy cows and contaminating milk; commercial household chemicals and cosmetics; lindane lice shampoos; workplace carcinogens; and lifestyle risks, such as the use of alcohol, tobacco, and dark hair dyes. Dr. Epstein also recommends that pre-menopausal women avoid mammograms, and that children and pregnant women limit their exposure to x-rays.

CONSULT YOUR PHYSICIAN BEFORE GETTING STARTED

Be sure to discuss all these detoxification options with a physician trained in these procedures, such as a naturopath or integrative medicine doctor. Ideally, your detoxification program should be conducted under a doctor's supervision. The major contraindications to detoxification are pregnancy and breastfeeding. However, because there are no routine or inexpensive tests to diagnose toxicity, nobody really knows how toxic they are or what the consequences of going on a rigorous detoxification program might be. In addition, toxins are notorious for hiding in fat cells. When fat cells break down to provide energy, they automatically release toxins. These toxins then circulate in the blood, making their way into the brain and all other body tissues. Symptoms of brain fog, irritability, anxiety, and even depression can accompany toxins flooding the brain. It is therefore highly rec-ommended that you seek guidance for your detoxification program to help you understand the difference between a "healing reaction" and a medical problem.

Once you have guidance on your detoxification program you can begin by squeezing half a lemon in some water and drinking that to begin your morning. Then do a regular Epsom salt bath, a sauna, or a steam bath. The key to detoxifying is to do it regularly. You and your doctor can make the rules for your detoxification, but make them you must, in order to stay healthy and vibrant in today's toxic world. Go about your detoxification slowly and deliberately, trying not to be overwhelmed by the immensity of the problem. As you begin to feel better when you go on a healthier diet and cut out the chemicals in your life, you will have more energy to tackle bigger issues. But remember to just take one step at a time.

Conclusion

Newspapers, magazines, and other publications run ads every day for the newest cures for various horrible and loathsome diseases. How is it that, despite hype like "Cancer's Magic Bullet Discovered," or "Perfect Cure for Heart Disease" and others, people are still getting sick? The reason is because neither diet, exercise, nor any other part of our lifestyle, are mentioned in the eight-page mailer from which those ads came. As a result of such short-sighted approaches, all common degenerative diseases are increasing around the world, especially heart disease, cancer, diabetes, arthritis, asthma and other respiratory conditions. And obesity is now recognized as a worldwide epidemic. People run from one healer to another looking for the answer to many of their symptoms. They deny that food and other lifestyle factors affect their lives, and they miss out on the right solutions. Some may worry about vaccinations, dental fillings, and the host of chemicals that invade our lives, but the biggest worry should be ongoing toxic intrusion from the cesspool of our intestines when our barriers are weakened.

We create our own diseases, something that should be readily apparent to you now that you have read this book. We ingest too much sugar, processed foods, and react badly to the stress in our life, so bad things happen. A starting point is to remove *all* sugar, wheat, and dairy from your diet, because I've been saying for twenty years that 80 percent of people with degenerative diseases who did this would get better. Writing this book has not changed my opinion. As the research shows, all three of these food culprits are linked to inflammation. Obese people are especially warned about these food classes, because they are also addictive and can cause disease.

Everything is related. Once one thing goes wrong with your health more things can go wrong. Allergies can show up first and then may become any nasty ailment your imagination can conjure up. Inflammation leads the way with most diseases. Homeostasis becomes the key to breaking this continuing cycle of disease, whether it is high blood pressure, heart disease, edema, or chronic fatigue.

A body in homeostasis is the building block of your health, so remove food allergies, remove abusive foods, and learn to change your stress from an obstacle to an opportunity. Don't eat in stressful situations. Be mindful of AGEs, free radicals, and chemicals. Make sure you do not have any low-grade infections anywhere in your body. Employ the food plans in Chapter 7 and your body will heal on the cheap. Inflammation will no longer be a problem.

Nothing happens for free, so forgive yourself when you fail, and resolve to do better next time. But don't forgive yourself to the point where no changes ever happen. Without homeostasis, no supplement or drug will help you. Health or disease, the choice is yours. You now have the information you need to choose wisely.

Glossary

AGEs. Sugar and protein that binds nonenzymatically in the body, producing glycated protein or advanced glycation end products (AGEs). Also called glycotoxins.

allergen. An antigenic substance capable of producing immediate type hypersensitivity reaction or a delayed reaction (allergy).

allergy. Allergies are inappropriate or exaggerated reactions of the immune system to substances that, in the majority of people, cause no symptoms. Symptoms of the allergic diseases may be caused by a food, chemicals, dust, pollen, or other substances.

anaphylactic shock. *See* anaphylaxis.

anaphylaxis or anaphylactic shock. A severe, frightening and life-threatening allergic reaction. The reaction, although rare, can occur after an insect sting or as a reaction to an injected or oral drug, a chemical, food, or inhalant.

angina. While this term is commonly interchanged with angina pectoris, a heart-related chest pain, it specifically refers to an inflammation of the throat characterized by spasmodic suffocation or suffocating pain.

angioedema. Large amounts of fluids in the blood vessels.

ankylosing spondylitis. A poly-arthritis involving the spine, which is characterized by progressive, painful stiffening of the joints and ligaments.

antigen. A protein marker on the surface of cells that identifies the cell as "self" or "non-self" (foreign). Antigens on "non-self" cells stimulate the production of antibodies to neutralize or destroy foreign invaders in the body (bacteria, fungi, viruses, yeasts, etc.).

171

antibody. A protein (also called an immunoglobulin) that is manufactured by lymphocytes (a type of white blood cell) to neutralize an antigen or foreign protein. Although many types of antibodies are protective, inappropriate or excessive formation of antibodies may lead to illness.

appendicitis. Inflammation of the appendix.

arrhythmia. An irregular heart beat.

arteriosclerosis. A term applied to a number of conditions involving thickening or hardening arteries, and/or arteries which have lost their elasticity.

asthma. Chronic, inflammatory lung disease characterized by recurrent breathing problems. When the air passages in asthmatic lungs get narrower, breathing becomes more difficult. Sometimes episodes of asthma are triggered by allergens, although infection, exercise, cold air and other factors are also important triggers.

atherosclerosis. The most common form of arteriosclerosis, characterized by the buildup of fatty deposits and cholesterol on the inner artery walls. In some cases calcium deposits may also form. As a result of atherosclerosis, blood vessels narrow, thicken, harden, and loose elasticity, blood flow decreases, and thrombosis, heart disease and stroke may result.

autoantibody. An antibody produced by B-cells in response to the immune system mistaking "self" antigens as foreign invaders in the body. Autoantibodies are the cause of autoimmune disease.

autoimmune disease. A condition in which the immune system mistakenly attacks the body's own organs and tissues.

B-cells. A type of white blood cells, which can produce antibody proteins necessary to fight off infections.

bronchitis. Inflammation of the bronchi (lung airways), resulting in persistent cough that produces considerable quantities of sputum (phlegm). Bronchitis is more common in smokers and in areas with high atmospheric pollution.

carcinogenic. Producing a malignant (cancerous) growth.

cardiomyopathy. A chronic disorder affecting the muscle of the heart, many times the cause is unknown.

celiac disease. A condition where the digestive tract fails to digest and absorb gliadin, a substance found in gluten, causing atrophy of the digestive and absorptive cells in the intestine.

chronic fatigue syndrome. Unexplained persistent or relapsing chronic fatigue that is of new or definite onset (i.e., not lifelong), is not the result of ongoing exertion, is not substantially alleviated by rest. It results in substantial reduction in previous levels of occupational, educational, social, or personal activities.

complement system. This series of molecules works together to perform many immune system functions. For example, the complement system helps to dissolve and remove immune complexes and to kill foreign cells.

conjunctivitis. Inflammation of the clear membrane that coats the inner lining of the eyelids and the outer surface of the eye.

coronary artery disease. The process by which coronary arteries become narrowed or completely clogged.

corticosteroid (corticoid, cortisone). Any steroid hormone made by the adrenal cortex, or made synthetically, which have powerful anti-inflammatory effects and are used to treat conditions involving inflammation.

C-reactive protein (CRP). A marker of inflammation in the bloodstream.

cytokines. Chemical substances that have varied effects on many cells of the body. For example, some cytokines can cause growth and activation of immune system cells and inflammation.

dermatitis. Inflammation of the skin or a rash caused by various substances of a chemical, animal or vegetable nature which a person can come in contact with or ingest.

digestive system. The group of organs that breaks down food into chemical components that the body can absorb and use for energy and for building and repairing cells and tissues.

edema. Swelling of tissue through increase of its (primarily) intercellular fluid content, due to passage of extra amounts of water out from capillaries.

ELISA. Blood test used to detect IgG antibodies to specific allergens.

emphysema. A chronic lung condition that affects the air sacs in the lungs (alveoli). It is characterized by shortness of breath, coughing, fatigue, loss of sleep, heart problems (endocarditis, inflammation of the lining of the heart cavity and valves), weight loss, and depression.

endogenous. Caused by factors inside the organism or system.

endotoxins. Chemicals synthesized to specifically initiate inflammation.

enzyme. A protein molecule produced by living organisms that catalyses chemical reactions of other substances without itself being destroyed or altered upon completion of the reactions.

eosinophils. A type of white blood cell that is particularly associated with parasitic infections and with hypersensitivity and allergic reactions.

gluten intolerance. Allergy to wheat, barley, rye, oats, spelt, and kamut.

glycotoxins. *See* AGEs.

histamine. A chemical present in cells throughout the body that is released during an allergic reaction. Histamine is one of the substances responsible for the symptoms of inflammation, and is the major reason for running of the nose, sneezing, and itching in allergic rhinitis. It also stimulates production of acid by the stomach and narrows the bronchi or airways in the lungs.

homeostasis. A balance of all body functions and systems. When homeostasis is impaired, the stage is set for disease.

hydrogenated fats. Fats that add extra hydrogen atoms used in margarines.

hyperkinetic. Hyperactivity, characterized by fast-paced or frenetic activity.

immune complex. A cluster of interlocking antigens and antibodies forming a large network of molecules.

immune system. A collection of cells and proteins that works to protect the body from potentially harmful, infectious microorganisms (microscopic life-forms), such as bacteria, viruses and fungi. The immune system plays a role in the control of cancer and other diseases, but also is the culprit in the phenomena of allergies, hypersensitivity, and the rejection of transplanted organs, tissues, and medical implants.

immunoglobulin. *See* antibody.

inflammation. A form of immune response that occurs in response to any form of bodily injury or insult, including physical trauma, infection, food allergies, exposure to chemicals or other environmental toxins, and extreme temperature. This response can cause redness, swelling, heat, and pain in a tissue if the bodily injury or insult remains chronic or unresolved.

interleukin. Proteins produced by lymphocytes, monocytes and various other cell types and are released by cells in response to antigenic and non-antigenic stimuli.

ischemic heart disease. An inadequate flow of blood to blood vessels causing restriction of the blood vessels.

kinins. Inflammatory mediators that cause dilation of blood vessels and altered vascular permeability.

leukotrienes. A group of chemicals that help regulate inflammatory reactions because of their ability to constrict blood vessels and attract various types of immune cells.

lifestyle. The manner in which we carry on our individual daily lives. Factors include our diet, exercise, stress management, recreation, and attitude toward life.

lymphocyte. A type of white blood cell of the immune system. T-cells and B-cells are lymphocytes that look similar under the microscope but have different functions.

macrophage. A type of white blood cell that functions as a patrol cell and engulfs and kills foreign infectious invaders.

mast cells. Play an important role in the body's allergic response. Mast cells are present in most body tissues, but are numerous in connective tissue. In an allergic response, an allergen stimulates the release of antibodies, which attach themselves to mast cells. Following subsequent allergen exposure, the mast cells release substances such as histamine into the tissue.

mediator. A substance released from cells as the result of the interaction of antigen with antibody.

microorganism. A microscopic organism, those of medical interest include bacteria, viruses, algae, fungi and protozoa.

myocardial infarction. Death of a segment of heart muscle, which follows interruption of its blood supply.

myocarditis. Acute or chronic inflammation of the heart.

neuron. A nerve encompassing the cell and the long fiber originating from the cell.

neuropeptides. Neurotransmitter with direct effect on the nervous system.

neurotransmitter. Chemical messenger that works throughout the body.

pericarditis. Acute or chronic inflammation of the membranous sac (pericardium), surrounding the heart.

probiotics. The living beneficial bacteria that support digestion as well as vaginal and urinary tract health.

prostaglandin. One of a group of hormone-like substances present in a wide variety of tissues and body fluids.

psycho-neuro-gastro-endrocrino-immunology. The study of the connection between the nerves, the mind, the digestive, endocrine, and immune system.

psychoneuroimmunology. The study of the connection between the mind and the immune system.

psychosocial. Psychological and social aspects; age, education, marital and related aspects of a person's history.

RAST. Blood test used to detect IgE antibodies to specific allergens.

rhinitis. Inflammation of the mucous membrane that lines the nose, often due to an allergy to pollen, dust, or other airborne substances. Seasonal allergic rhinitis also is known as "hay fever," a disorder which causes sneezing, itching, a runny nose, and nasal congestion. Rhinitis can be caused by food and chemicals.

sinusitis. Inflammation of the membrane lining the facial sinuses, often caused by bacterial or viral infection, food or chemical allergy.

stroke. Condition due to the lack of oxygen to the brain due to interrupted blood flow, caused by a blood clot or blood vessel bursting, which may lead to reversible or irreversible paralysis, coma, speech problems, and dementia.

T-cell. A type of lymphocyte. T-cells have T-cell receptors and, sometimes, co-stimulatory molecules on their cell surfaces. The T-cell helps to orchestrate the immune system and can issue "orders" for other cells to make cytokines and chemokines.

thrombophlebitis. Inflammation of a vein associated with thrombus formation, blood clot.

References

Introduction

1. Libby, P. "The Fire Within." *Scientific American*. May 2002: 48–55.

Chapter 1

1. "Clinical Aspects of Acute Inflammation." http://medweb.bham.ac.uk/http/mod/3/1/a/clinical.html.

2. "Chronic Inflammation." http://medweb.bham.ac.uk/http/depts/path/Teaching/FOUNDAT/CHRONINF/chronic.html.

3. Incao, P.F. "Vaccine Information" www.mercola.com/1999/Aug/22/vaccine_information.html

Buttram, H.E. "Vaccine Scene 2001: Update and Overview." Part 1 and 2, April 16, 2002. www.mercola.com/2001/Jun/9/vaccine_update.htm.

4. Koh, K. K., et al. "Statin Attunuates Increase in C-Reactive Protein During Estrogen Replacement Therapy in Postmenopausal Women." *Circulation*. Dec 10, 2002;106(24):198–199.

5. Hellermann, G., et al. "Mechanism of Cigarette Smoke Condensate-induced Acute Inflammatory Response in Human Bronchial Epithelial Cells." *Respir Res.* 2002;3:22.

6. Repka-Ramirez, S., et al. "Cytokines in Nasal Lavage Fluids from Acute Sinusitis, Allergic Rhinitis, and Chronic Fatigue Syndrome Subjects." *Allergy Asthma Proc.* May–Jun 2002;23(3):185–90.

7. Starr, C., "Infections and Heart Disease." *Hippocrates Magazine.* www.hippocrates.com/archives...y2001/01departments/01horizon.html.

8. Ghosh, S. et al. "New Approach to Thwarting Inflammation." *Science.* September 1, 2000 & www.hhmi.org/news//ghosh.html.

Chapter 2

1. Cannon, W. B. *The Wisdom of the Body*. (New York: Norton, 1932. 2nd edition, 1939).

2. Kushner, I. "Semantics, Inflammation, Cytokines, and Common Sense." *Cytokine & Growth Factor Reviews*. 1998;9(3/4):191–196.

3. Page, M. and Abrams, L. H. Jr. *Your Body Is Your Best Doctor*. (New Canaan, CT: Keats Publishing, 1972).

4. Albrecht, W. A. *The Albrecht Papers*. (Kansas City, KS: Acre, 1975).

5. Analytical Research Labs Inc. 2338 West Royal Palm Road, #F, Phoenix AR 85021.

6. Ashmead, D. *Chelated Mineral Nutrition*. (Huntington Beach, CA: International Institute of Natural Health Sciences, Inc., 1979).

7. Ratner, B. G. and Gruehl, H. L. "Passage of Native Proteins through the Normal Gastrointestinal Wall." *Journal of Clinical Investigation*. 1934;13;517.

Warshaw, A. L., et al. "Protein Uptake by the Intestine: Evidence for Absorption of Intact Macromolecules." *Gastroenterology*. 1974;66:987.

8. Philpott, W. *Brain Allergies*. (New Canaan, CT: Keats Publishing Inc., 1980).

9. Hevman, M. "Symposium on Dietary Influences on Mucosal Immunity— How Dietary Antigens Access the Mucosal Immune System." *Proc Ntitr Soc*. 2001 Nov,60(4):419–426.

10. Philpott, W. *Brain Allergies*. 104.

11. Baker, B. "Patient History Often Fails to Uncover Allergies." *Skin & Allergy News*. April, 1997; 11.

12. Philpott, W. *Brain Allergies*. 104.

Chapter 3
Food Allergy

1. Rothenberg, M., et. al. "A Pathological Function for Eotaxin and Eosinophils in Eosinophilic Gastrointestinal Inflammation." *Nature Immunology*. 2001; 2: 353–60.

2. Forman, R. *How to Control Your Allergies* (Larchmont Books, New York, 1979).

3. Gaby, A. "The Role of Hidden Food Allergy in Chronic Disease." *Alt Med Rev*. 1998; 3 (2): 90–100.

4. Edwards, T. "Failure to Thrive." *Clinical & Environmental Allergy*. 1995; 25: 16–19.

Berger, S. *Immune Power Diet*. (New American Library, New York, 1985).

5. Alpha Nutrition Center, Food Allergy Center. www.nutramed.com/foodallergy/index.htm.

6. Braly, James, MD. "Dr. Braly's Allergy Relief, the Natural Way." www.drbralyallergyrelief.com/igg.html.

7. Walker, W. "IgG Blood Print Determination of Adverse Responses to Food." *Townsend Letter for Doctors.* July 1991; 566–570.

Stevens, W.J., and Bridts, C.H. "IgG-containing Circulating Immune Complexes in Patients with Asthma and Rhinitis." *Journal of Allergy and Clinical Immunology.* 1979; 63: 297.

8. Philpott, W. and Kalita, D.K. *Victory Over Diabetes.* 22–24. (New Canaan, CT: Keats Publishing Inc., 1983.)

9. Calabrese, D. "Food Allergies and Addiction." www.enviromed.org

10. Rothenberg, M.E. *Nature Immunology.* April 2001.

11. Rothenberg, M., et al. "A Pathological Function for Eotaxin and Eosinophils in Eosinophilic Gastrointestinal Inflammation." *Nature Immunology.* 2001; 2: 353–360.

12. *Ibid.*

13. Dieth, E.A. "The Role of Intestinal Barrier Failure and Bacterial Translocation in the Development of Systemic Infection and Multiple Organ Failure." *Arch Surgery.* 1990; 125: 403–4.

14. Schwarz, B., et al. "Intestinal Ischemic Reperfusion Syndrome: Pathophysiology, Clinical Significance, Therapy." (In German). *Wien Klin Wochenschr.* July 30, 1999; 111 (14): 539–48.

15. Bjarnson, I., et al. "The Leaky Gut of Alcoholism. Possible Route for Entry of Toxic Compounds." *Lancet.* 1984; 1: 179–82.

16. Read, N.W. "Food and Hypersensitivity in Functional Dyspepsia." *Gut.* July 2002; 51 (Supp 1:I): 50–53.

Environmental Allergies

17. "A Report on Multiple Chemical Sensitivities (MCS)." www. health.gov/environment/mcs/i.htm.

18. Pope, C. A. 3rd. "Lung Cancer, Cardiopulmonary Mortality, and Long-term Exposure to Fine Particulate Air Pollution." *JAMA.* Mar 6, 2002;287: 1132–1141.

Bircher, A. J, et al. "IgE to Food Allergens are Highly Prevalent in Patients Allergic to Pollens, With and Without Symptoms of Food Allergy." *Clin Exp Allergy.* 1994;24:367–374.

19. Eysink, P. E., et al."Do Levels of Immunoglobulin G Antibodies to Foods Predict the Development of Immunoglobulin E Antibodies to Cat, Dog And/or Mite?" *Clin Exp Allergy.* Apr 2002;32(4):556–562.

20. Pastorello, E. "Evaluation of Allergic Etiology in Perennial Rhinitis." *Annals of Allergy.* Dec 1985;55:854–856.

21. Calkhoven, P.G., et al. "Relationship Between IgG1 and IgG4 Antibodies to Foods and the Development of IgE Antibodies to Inhalant Allergens. Increased Levels of IgE Antibodies to Foods in Children Who Subsequently Develop IgE Antibodies to Inhalant Allergens." *Clin Exp Allergy.* Jan 1991;21:99–107.

22. Mercola, J. www.mercola.com.

23. Roberts, G., Golder N. and Lack G. "Bronchial Challenges with Aerosolized Food in Asthmatic, Food-allergic Children." *Allergy.* 2002;57(8):713–717.

24. Spannhake, E. W. "Synergism Between Rhinovirus Infection and Oxidant Pollutant Exposure Enhances Airway Epithelial Cell Cytokine Production." *Environ Health Perspect.* Jul 2002; 110(7):665–670.

25. Race, Sharla. "Amines in Food." http://tigmor.com/food/library/articles/am_food.htm.

26. Feingold Association of America. www.feingold.org/home.html.

27. Terrell, T., et al. "Identifying Exercise Allergies: Exercise-Induced Anaphylaxis and Cholinergic Urticaria." *Physical and Sportsmedicine.* 24:11, November 1996. www.physsportsmed.com/issues/nov_96/terre;/htm.

28. Ikonomidis, I., et al. "Increased Proinflammatory Cytokines in Patients with Chronic Stable Angina and Their Reduction by Aspirin." *Circulation* Aug 24, 1999;100:793–798.

Sheth, T. "Comparison of the Effects of Omapatrilat and Lisinopril on Circulating Neurohormones and Cytokines in Patients with Chronic Heart Failure." *Am J Cardiol.* Sep 1, 2002;90(5):496–500.

29. "Profile of Patients with Chemical Injury and Sensitivity," *Environmental Health Perspectives.* 1997;105 (Suppl 2):417–436.

Chapter 4

AGEs

1. Bunn, F. and Higgins, P. J. "Reaction of Monosaccharides with Protein: Possible Evolutionary Significance." *Science.* Jul 10, 1981;213.

2. Economic Research Service. U.S. Department of Agriculture. www.ers.usda.gov/brfiefing/sugar/background.htm.

3. Cerami, C., et al. "Tobacco Smoke Is a Source of Toxic Reactive Glycation Products." *Proc Natl Acad Sci USA.* Dec 9, 1997;25(139):15–20.

4. Saari, J. and Dahlen, G. "Dietary Copper Deficiency Causes Elevation of Early and Advanced Glycation End-Products." U.S. Department of Agriculture. www.nps.ars.usda.gov/publications/publications.htm?SEQ_NO_115=101255.

5. Furth, A. and Harding, J. "Why Sugar Is Bad For You." *New Scientist.* Sep 23, 1989;44.

6. *Estimated Annual Production and Consumption of Soft Drinks.* Washington, DC: Soft Drink Association, 1986.

7. Szymanska, U. and Boratynski, J. "Protein Glycation–Clinical and Chemical Aspects." *Postepy Hig Med Dosw.* 1999;53(5):689–703.

8. "Advanced Glycation End-Products (AGEs) and Cataract—Distribution in Different Types of Cataract." www.dog.org/2001/abstract_german/Dawczynski_e.htm.

9. Ishibashi, T., et al. "Advanced Glycation End Products in Age-related Macular Degeneration." *Arch Ophthalmol.* Dec 1998;116(12):1629–1632.

10. Vlassara, H., et al. "Inflammatory Mediators Are Induced by Dietary Glycotoxins, a Major Risk Factor for Diabetic Angiopathy." *Proc Natl Acad Sci USA.* Nov 26, 2002;99:15596–15601.

11. MacLennan, A. "Identification of the Advanced Glycation End Products N-epsilon-carboxymethyllysine in the Synovial Tissue of Patients with Rheumatoid Arthritis." *Annals of the Rheumatic Diseases* (ARD Online). Sep 12, 2002.

12. Tabaton, M., et al. "Is Amyloid Beta-protein Glycated in Alzheimer's Disease?" *Neuroreport.* 1997; 8(4):907–909.

13. Furth, A.J. "Glycated Proteins in Diabetes."*Br J Biomed Sci.* Sep 1997; 54(3):192–200.

14. Dominic, S. C., et al. "Advanced Glycation End Products: a Nephrologist's Perspective." *Am J Kidney Dis.* 2000;35(3):365–380.

15. Krajoviová-Kudláková, M. *Physiol. Res.* 2002;51:313–316.

16. Mullarkey, C. J., et al."Free Radical Generation by Early Glycation Products: A Mechanism for Accelerated Atherogenesis in Diabetes." *Biochem Biophys Res Commun.* Dec 31, 1990;173(3):932–939.

17. Mottram, D. S., et al. "Acrylamide Is Formed in the Maillard Reaction." *Nature.* Oct 3, 2002;419(6906):448–449.

Stadler, R. H. "Food Chemistry: Acrylamide from Maillard Reaction Products." *Nature.*

18. Tareke, E., et al. "Analysis of Acrylamide, a Carcinogen Formed in Heated Foodstuffs." *J Agric Food Chem.* Aug 14, 2002;50(17):4998–5006.

19. Flick, F. "Experts Launch Action on Acrylamide in Staple Foods." *BMJ.* Jul 20, 2002;325:120.

20. Vlassara, H., et al. "Inflammatory Mediators Are Induced by Dietary Glycotoxins, a Major Risk Factor for Diabetic Angiopathy." *Proc. Natl. Acad. Sci. USA.* Nov 26, 2002; 99(24): 15596–15601.

21. Mirkin, G. "Advanced Glycation End Products." www.drmirkin.com/ archive.

22. Cerami, C., et al. "Tobacco Smoke Is a Source of Toxic Reactive Glycation Products." *Proc Natl Acad Sci USA.* Dec 9, 1997;94(25):13915–13920.

23. Dickerson, T. and Janda, K. "A Previously Undescribed Chemical Link Between Smoking and Metabolic Disease." *PNAS.* Nov 12, 2002;99(23):15084–15088.

Free Radicals

24. Harmon, D. "Defeating Free Radicals: The Key to Longevity." Chapter 2 *Anti-aging Book.* www.renewalresearch.com/book/defeating_free_radicals.html.

25."The Free Radical Theory." www.nutritionaltest.com/freeradical.html.

26. Oteiza, P. I., et al. "Zinc Deficiency Induces Oxidative Stress and Ap-1 Activation in 3t3 Cells." *Free Radic Biol Med.* Apr 1, 2000;28(7):1091–1099.

27. Harmon, D. "Defeating Free Radicals: The Key to Longevity." Chapter 2 *Antiaging Book*. www.renewalresearch.com/book/defeating_free_radicals.html.

28. Capone, G. "Evidence for Increased Mitochondrial Superoxide Production in Down Syndrome." *Life Sci*. May 3, 2002;70(24):2885–2895.

Psychological Stress

29. Edwards, T. "Failure to Thrive." *Clinical & Environmental Allergy*. 1995; 25:16–19.

30. Mandell, M. *Dr. Mandell's 5 Day Allergy Relief System*. (New York: Thomas Y. Crowell, Publishers, 1976).

31. Berger, S. *Immune Power Diet*. (New York: New American Library, 1985).

32. Philpott, W. and Kalita, D.K. *Brain Allergies*.

33. Theoharides, T. C., et al."Stress-induced Intracranial Mast Cell Degranulation:A Corticotropin-releasing Hormone-mediated Effect." *Endocrinology*. Dec 1995;136(12):5745–5750.

34. Rothenberg, M., et al. "A Pathological Function for Eotoxin and Eosinophils in Eosinophilic Gastrointestinal Inflammation." *Nature Immunology*. 2001;2: 353–360.

35. *Ibid*.

36. Philpott, *Brain Allergies*. 12.

37. Philpott, W. H. and Kalita, D. K.. *Victory over Diabetes*, 60.

38. Mandell, 203.

39. Mandell, 109.

40. Philpott, *Brain Allergies*.

41. Marshall, P. S. "Effects of Seasonal Allergic Rhinitis on Fatigue Levels and Mood." *Psychosom Med*. Jul–Aug 2002;64(4):684–691.

42. Dickey, L. D. (ed.), Randolph, T. G. "Biological Dietetic." *Clinical Ecology*. (Springfield MA: Charles C. Thomas, 1976) 107–121.

43. Mackarness, R. *Eating Dangerously*. (New York: Harcourt, 1976).

44. Lundberg, A. "Psychiatric Aspects of Air Pollution." *Otolaryngol Head Neck Surg*. Feb 1996;114(2):227–231.

45. Badgley, L. "Immune System: Nature's Intelligence Confronts Modern Technology." *International Journal of Holistic Health and Medicine*. July 1985;3(4):26.

46. "Depression and Mood Disorders." www.gsdl.com/assessments/finddisease/depression/.

47. Black, P. H. "Immune System-central Nervous System Interactions: Effect and Immunomodulatory Consequences of Immune System Mediators on the Brain." *Antimicrob Agents Chemother*. Jan 1994;38(1):7–12.

48. Miller, G. E., et al. "Chronic Psychological Stress and the Regulation of Pro-Inflammatory Cytokines: A Glucocorticoid-Resistance Model." *Health Psychology*. 2002; 21 (6): 531–541.

49. Raison, C. L. and Miller, A.H. "The Neuroimmunology of Stress and Depression." *Semin Clin Neuropsychiatry.* Oct 2001;6(4):277–294.

50. Cernak, I., et al. "Alterations in Magnesium and Oxidative Status During Chronic Emotional Stress." *Magnes Res.* Mar 2000;13(1):29–36.

51. Mandell, 109.

Chapter 5
Alzheimer's Disease

1. Hull, M., et al. "Pathways of Inflammatory Activation in Alzheimer's Disease: Potential Targets for Disease Modifying Drugs." *Curr Med Chem.* Jan 2002;9(1):83–88.

2. Aisen, P. S. "The Potential of Anti-inflammatory Drugs for the Treatment of Alzheimer's Disease." *Lancet Neurol.* Sep 2002;1 (5):279–284.

3. Lovell, M. A., et al. "Elevated Thiobarbituric Acid-Reactive Substances and Antioxidant Enzyme Activity in the Brain in Alzheimer's Disease." *Neurology.*1995;451:1594–1601.

4. Perry, G., et al. "Reactive Oxygen Species Mediate Cellular Damage in Alzheimer Disease." *JAD.* Mar 1998;1(1):45–55.

5. Butterfield, D. A., et al. "Amyloid Beta-peptide and Amyloid Pathology Are Central to the Oxidative Stress and Inflammatory Cascades under Which Alzheimer's Disease Exists." *J Alzheimers Dis.* Jun 2002;4(3):193–201.

6. Aisen, 279–284.

7. Verbeek, M. M., et al. "Inflammatory Mechanisms in the Pathogenesis of Alzheimer's Disease." *Tijdschr Gerontol Geriatr.* Oct 28, 1997;(5):213–218.

8. Christopher, C. W., et al. "Retrograde Degeneration of Neurite Membrane Structural Integrity of Nerve Growth Cones Following in Vitro Exposure to Mercury." *NeuroReport.* 2001;2(4):733–737.

9. Connor, J. R., et al. "Is Hemochromatosis a Risk Factor for Alzheimer's Disease?" *J Alzheimers Dis.* Oct 2001;3(5):471–477.

10. Laurin, D., et al. "Physical Activity and Risk of Cognitive Impairment and Dementia in Elderly Persons." *Archives of Neurology.* Mar 2001;58:498–504.

11. Friedland, R. P., et al. "Patients with Alzheimer's Disease Have Reduced Activities in Midlife Compared with Health Control-group Members." *Proc Natl Acad Sci USA.* Mar 13, 2001;98(6):3440–3445.

Blood Sugar Problems

1. OHSU Health. "Diabetes Statistics." www.ohsuhealth.com/diabetes/ stats.asp.

2. Vaarala, O. "The Gut Immune System and Type 1 Diabetes." *Annals NYAS.* 2002;958:39–46.

3. Philpott, W. and Kalita, D. K. *Victory over Diabetes.* (New Canaan, CT: Keats Publishing, Inc., 1980)24–26.

4. Becker, D. J., et al. "Prevention of Type 1 Diabetes: Is Now the Time?" *J Clin Endocrinol Metab.* 2000; 85: 498–506.

5. Overton, S., 62nd Annual Meeting of the American Diabetes Association in San Francisco CA; June 14–18, 2002.

6. Philpott and Kalita, *Victory over Diabetes.*

7. *Ibid.*

8. Philpott and Kalita, *Victory over Diabetes.*

9. Pradhan, A. D., et al. "C-reactive Protein, Interleukin 6, and Risk of Developing Type 2 Diabetes Mellitus." JAMA. Jul 18, 2001;286(3):261–274.

10. *Ibid.*

11. Philpott and Kalita, *Victory over Diabetes.*

12. Paolisso, G. and Giugliano, D. "Oxidative Stress and Insulin Action: Is There a Relationship?" *Diabetologia.* 1996;39;357–363.

13. Vlassara, H., et al. "Inflammatory Mediators Are Induced by Dietary Glycotoxins, a Major Risk Factor for Diabetic Angiopathy." *Proc Natl Acad Sci USA.* Nov 26,2002;99:15596–15601.

14. Thorand, B., et al. "C-reactive Protein as a Predictor for Incident Diabetes Mellitus among Middle-aged Men: Results from the Monica Augsburg Cohort Study, 1984–1998." *Arch Intern Med.* Jan 13, 2003;163(1):93–99.

15. Levine, S. "Food Addiction, Food Allergy and Overweight." www.springboard4health.com/notebook/health_food_addiction.html.

16. Correspondence with Jeffrey Moss, Oct 21, 2002.

17. Trevisan, M., et al. "Syndrome X and Mortality: a Population-based Study." *J Epidemiol.* Nov 15, 1998;148(10):958–966.

18. Meigs, J. B. "Epidemiology of the Metabolic Syndrome." *Am J Manag Care.* Sep 8, 2002 (11 Suppl):S283–92; quiz S293–6.

19. McAuley, K. A., et al. "Diagnosing Insulin Resistance in the General Population." *Diabetes Care.* 2000;24(3):460–464.

20. Timar, O., et al. "Metabolic Syndrome X: A Review." *Canadian Journal of Cardiology.* June 2000;16 (6):779–789.

21. Denke, M.A. "Metabolic Syndrome." *Curr Atheroscler Rep.* Nov 4, 2002; 6:444–447.

Cancer

1. Moss, R. "The War on Cancer." *Townsend Letter for Doctors and Patients.* Nov 2001:220:22–23.

2. O'Byrne, K. J., and Dalgleish, A.G. "Chronic Immune Activation and Inflammation as the Cause of Malignancy." *Br J Cancer.* Aug 17, 2001;85(4):473–483.

3. *Ibid.*

4. Stein, R. "Innflammation May Spur Diseases: Cancer, Even Alzheimer's, May Begin with Body's First Defense." *Washington Post.* www.msnbe.com/ news/ 873592.asp?0cv=CB20.

5. Ohshima. H. "Endogenous Cancer Risk Factors." www.iarc.fr/pageroot/UNITS/ECR.HTM.

6. Hietanen, E., et al. "Diet and Oxidative Stress in Breast, Colon, and Prostate Cancer Patients: a Case-Control Study." *Eur J Clin Nutr.* 48(8) 575–586.

7. Cerutti, P., et al. "The Role of the Cellular Antioxidant Defense in Oxidant Carcinogenesis." *Environmental Health Perspectives.* 1994;102(10):123–130.

8. Hristozov, D., et al. "Evaluation of Oxidative Stress in Patients with Cancer." *Archives of Physiology and Biochemistry.* 2001;109(4):331–336.

9. Yamamoto, Y., et al. "Advanced Glycation Endproducts-Receptor Interactions Stimulate the Growth of Human Pancreatic Cancer Cells through the Induction of Platelet-Derived Growth Factor-B." *Biochemical and Biophysical Research Communications.* May 24, 1996;22(3):700–705.

10. Hiroki, H., et al. "Expression of Receptors for Advanced Glycation End-products (Rage) Is Closely Associated with the Invasive and Metastatic Activity of Gastric Cancer." *Journal of Pathology.* 2002;192(2):163–170.

11. McWhorter, W. P. "Allergy and Risk of Cancer: A Prospective Study Using NHANESI (First National Health and Nutrition Examination Survey) Followup Data." *Cancer.* 1988;62:451.

12. Shils, M. E. And Goodhart, R. S. "Nutrition and Neoplasia." *Modern Nutrition in Health and Disease.* (Philadelphia: Lea & Febiger, 1980)1177.

13. Catassi, C., et al. "Risk of Non-hodgkin Lymphoma in Celiac Disease."*JAMA.* 2002;287:1413–1419.

14. Mercola, J. "Allergies & Weight May Play Role In Lymphoma." www.mercola.com/1999/aug/15/allergies_and_weight_in_lymphoma.htm.

Candida

1. www.health-diets.net/healthsearch/calorie.htm.

2. "Questions about Candidiasis" http://ibscrohns.about.com/cs/candida/a/candidiasisfaq_2.htm.

Canker Sores and Mouth Ulcers

1. Thomas, H. C., et al. "Food Antibodies in Oral Disease: A Study of Serum Antibodies to Food Proteins in Aphthous Ulceration and Other Oral Diseases." *J Clin Pathol.* May 1973; 26(5):371–374.

2. Wright, A., et al. "Food Allergy or Intolerance in Severe Recurrent Aphthous Ulceration of the Mouth." *Br Med J* (Clin Res Ed). May 10, 1986;292(6530): 1237–1238.

3. Nolan, A. "Recurrent Aphthous Ulceration and Food Sensitivity." *J Oral Pathol Med.* Nov 20, 1991(10):473–475.

4. Wray, D. "Gluten-sensitive Recurrent Aphthous Stomatitis." *Dig Dis Sci.* Aug 1981: 26(8):737–740.

5. "Food Allergy and Oral Ulcerations." http://altmedicine.about.com/library/weekly/aa120601a.htm?terms=+food+allergies.

6. Wright, A., et al. "Food Allergy or Intolerance in Severe Recurrent Aphthous Ulceration of the Mouth." *Br Med J.* 1986;292:1237–1238.

Cystic Fibrosis

1. Konstan, M. W. "Bronchoalveolar Lavage Findings in Cystic Fibrosis Patients with Stable, Clinically Mild Lung Disease Suggest Ongoing Infection and Inflammation. *Am J Respir Crit Care Med.*1994;150:448–454.

2. Lucarelli, et al. "Food Allergy in Cystic Fibrosis." *Minerva Pediatr.* 1994;46(12):543–548.

3. Vazquez Cordero, C., et al. "Significance of IgG Serum Levels in Cystic Fibrosis." *An Esp Pediatr.* 1988;28(4):321–324.

4. Murali, P. S., et al. "Immune Response to Aspergillus Fumigatus and Pseudomonas Aeruginosa Antigens in Cystic Fibrosis and Allergic Bronchopulmonary Aspergillosis." *Chest.* 1994; 106(2): 349–352.

5. Birrer, P., et al. "Protease-antiprotease Imbalance in the Lungs of Children with Cystic Fibrosis." *Am J Respir Crit Care Med.* 1994;150:207–221.

Epilepsy

1. Frediani, T., et al. "Allergy and Childhood Epilepsy: A Close Relationship?" *Acta Neurologica Scandinavica.* 2001;104(6):349–335.

2. Kinsman, S. L., et al. "Efficacy of the Ketogenic Diet for Intractable Seizure Disorders: Review of 58 Cases." *Epilepsia.*1992;33:1132–1136.

3. Sudha, K., et al. "Oxidative Stress and Antioxidants in Epilepsy." *Clin Chim Acta.* Jan 2001;303(1–2):19–24.

4. Jiang, D., et al. "Chronic Brain Oxidation in a Glutathione Peroxidase Knockout Mouse Model Results in Increased Resistance to Induced Epileptic Seizures." *Exp Neurol.* Aug 2000;164(2):257–268.

5. Weber, K., et al. "Distribution of Advanced Glycation End Products in the Cerebellar Neurons of Dogs." *Brain Res.* Apr 27, 2002;791(1–2):11–7.

Food Allergy, Eating Disorders

1. Selye, H. *The Stress of Life.* (San Francisco, CA: McGraw-Hill,1978).

2. Mandell, p 108.

3. Mandell, p.109.

4. McGee, C. *How To Survive Modern Technology.* (New Canaan, CT: Keats Pub, 1980).

5. Volkow, N., et al. "Nonhedonic Food Motivation in Humans Involves Dopamine in the Dorsal Striatum and Methylphenidate Amplifies This Effect." *Synapse.* 44:2002:175–180.

6. Colantuoni, C., et al. "Evidence That Intermittent, Excessive Sugar Intake Causes Endogenous Opioid Dependence." *Obes Res.* Jun 2002;10(6):478–488.

7. Philpott, W, *Brain Allergies.*

8. Levine, Stephen. "Food Addiction, Food Allergy, and Overweight." www.springboard4health.com/notebook/health_food_addiction.ht.

9. Genet, P. et al. "Anorexic forms of celiac syndromes." *Ann Med Interne (Paris).* Mar 1972;123(3):237–40.

10. Johnson, J. G., et al. "Eating Disorders During Adolescence and the Risk for Physical and Mental Disorders During Early Adulthood." *Arch Gen Psychiatry.* Jun 2002;59(6):545–52.

Headaches

1. "Cluster Headaches." http://familydoctor.org/handouts/035.html.

2. Hadjivassiliou, M. "Headache and CNS White Matter Abnormalities Associated with Gluten Sensitivity." *Neurology.* February 2001;56:385–388.

3. Mansfield, I. E. "Food Allergy and Adult Migraine." *Annals of Allergy.* 1985; special issue 55:126.

4. Egger, J. et al. "Oligoantigenic Diet Treatment of Children with Epilepsy and Migraine." *J Pediatr.* 1989;114(1):51.

5. Grant, E. C. "Food Allergies and Migraine." *Lancet.* May 5, 1979; 5;1(8123): 966–969.

6. Ikeda, Y. "Headache: Direct Superoxide Scavenging Activity of Nonsteroidal Anti-inflammatory Drugs: Determination by Electron Spin Resonance Using the Spin Trap Method." *Journal of Head and Face Pain.* Feb 2001;41(2)138.

7. Sharma, V. P. "Tips for Chronic Stress Headaches." www.mindpub.com/art434.htm.

8. *Ibid.*

Heartburn

1. Rothenberg, M. "Cinciinati Researcher Uncovers Allergy/Reflux Link-Study Has Signifivant Treatment Implications." Dec. 27, 2002. www.cincinnatichildrens.org/about/news/release/2000/12-allergy-reflux.htm.

Heart Disease

1. Ventura, H. O. "Rudolph Virchow and Cellular Pathology." www.clinicalcardiology.org/briefs/200007briefs/cc23-550.profiles_virchow.html.

Rifai, N. and Ridker, P. M. "Inflammatory Markers and Coronary Heart Disease." *Curr Opin Lipidol.* Aug 2002;13(4):383–389.

2. Young, J. L. and Libby, P. "Cytokines in the Pathogenesis of Atherosclerosis." *Thromb Haemost.* Oct 2002;88(4):554–567.

American Heart Association. "Inflammation, Heart Disease, and Stroke: The Role of C-Reactive Protein." www.americanheart.org/Heart_and_Stroke_A_Z_Guide/inflamm.html.

3. "Protein Test Detects Heart Attack Risk." Heart Attack Center. www.heart1. com/attack/mainstory.cfm/45.

4. Rea, W. J. "Environmentally Triggered Thrombophlebitis." *Ann Allergy.* Aug 1976;37:101–109.

5. "AHA/ACC Scientific Statement: Assessment of Cardiovascular Risk by Use of Multiple-Risk-Factor Assessment Equations." *Circulation.* Oct 1, 1999;100: 1481–1492.

6. Caliguri, G. "Immune System Activation Follows Inflammation in Unstable Angina: Pathogenetic Implications." *J Am Coll Cardiol.* Nov 1, 1998;32:1295–1304.

7. Yudkin, J. and Eisa, O. "Dietary Sucrose and Oestradiol Concentration in Young Men." *Ann Nutr Metab.* 1988;32(2):53–55.

8. Liu, S., et al. "Relation Between a Diet with a High Glycemic Load and Plasma Concentrations of High-sensitivity C-reactive Protein in Middle-aged Women." *Am J Clin Nutr.* Mar 2002; 75(3):492–498.

9. Patel, P., et al. "Association of Helicobacter Pylori and Chlamydia Pneumoniae Infections with Coronary Heart Disease and Cardiovascular Risk Factors." *British Medical Journal.* 311; 1996:11–14.

10. Muhlestein, J.B., et al. "Increased Incidence of Chlamydia Species within the Coronary Arteries of Patients with Symptomatic Atherosclerotic Verses Other Forms of Cardiovascular Disease." *Journal of the American College of Cardiology.* 1996; 27:1555–1561.

11. Espinola-Klein, C. " Impact of Infectious Burden on Extent and Long-term Prognosis of Atherosclerosis." *Circulation.* Jan 1, 2002;105(1):15–21.

12. Siskovich, D., et al. "Interest in Link Between Inflammation and Heart Disease." American Heart Association." www.newswise.com/articles/2000/11/ INFLAM.HRT.html.

13. Stone, A. F., et al. "Effect of Treatment for Chlamydia Pneumoniae and Helicobacter Pylori on Markers of Inflammation and Cardiac Events in Patients with Acute Coronary Syndromes: South Thames Trial of Antibiotics in Myocardial Infarction and Unstable Angina." *Circulation.* Sep 3 2002;106(10):1219–1223.

14. Chae, C. U., et al. "Blood Pressure and Inflammation in Apparently Healthy Men." *Hypertension.* Sep 2001;38:399–403.

15. Grant, E. C. "Food Allergies and Migraine." *Lancet.* May 5, 1979; 5;1(8123): 966–969.

16. Sesso, H.D., et al. "C-Reactive Protein and the Risk of Developing Hypertension." *JAMA.* Dec. 10, 2003; 290 (22): 2945–51.

17. Caligiuri, G. "Immune System Activation Follows Inflammation in Unstable Angina: Pathogenetic Implications." *Journal of the American College of Cardiology.* November 1, 1998;32:1295–1304.

18. Rea, W. J. "Environmentally Triggered Cardiac Desease." *Ann Allergy.* Apr 1978;40(4):243–251.

19. Kanauchi, M., et al. "Advanced Glycation End Produces in Nondiabetic Patients with Coronary Artery Disease." *Diabetes Care.* 2001;24:1620–1623.

20. Ridker, P. M. "Comparison of C-Reactive Protein and Low-Density Lipopro-

tein Cholesterol Levels in the Prediction of First Cardiovascular Events." *N Engl J Med.* Nov 14, 2002;347(20):1557–1565.

21. Vlassara, H., et al. "Inflammatory Mediators Are Induced by Dietary Glyco-toxins, a Major Risk Factor for Diabetic Angiopathy."*Proc. Natl. Acad. Sci. USA,* Nov 26, 2002;99(24)15596–15601.

22. Cross, C. E., et al. "Oxygen Radicals and Human Disease." *Ann Int Med.* 1987;107: 526–545.

23. Tracy, R. P. "Inflammation in Cardiovascular Disease: Cart, Horse, or Both?" *Circulation.* May 26, 1998;97:2000.

24. Liu, Y. "Overtime Work, Insufficient Sleep, and Risk of Non-fatal Acute Myocardial Infarction in Japanese Men." *Occup Environ Med.* Jul 2002; 59(7):447–451.

Inflammatory Bowel Disease and Celiac Disease

1. Hunter, J. O., et al. "A Review of the Role of the Gut Microflora in Irritable Bowel Syndrome and the Effects of Probiotics." *Br J Nutr.* Sep 2002;88 (Suppl 1):67–72.

2. Zar, S., et al. "Food Hypersensitivity and Irritable Bowel Syndrome." *Alimentary Pharmacology and Therapeutics.* April 2001;15(4)439.

3. Wright, R. and Truelove, S. C. "Circulating Antibodies to Dietary Proteins in Ulcerative Colitis." *British Medical Journal.* 1965;2:142.

4. Zar, S., et al. "Role of Food Hypersensitivity in Irritable Bowel Syndrome." *Minerva Med.* Oct 2002;93(5):403–412.

5. Goldstein, R., et al. "Carbohydrate Malabsorption and the Effect of Dietary Restriction on Symptoms of Irritable Bowel Syndrome and Functional Bowel Complaints." *Isr Med Assoc J.* Aug 2000:8:583–587.

6. Hart, A. and Kamm, M. A. "Mechanisms of Initiation and Perpetuation of Gut Inflammation by Stress." *Alimentary Pharmacology & Therapeutics.* 2001;16 (12):2017.

7. Maxwell, P. R., et al. "Antibiotics Increase Functional Abdominal Symptoms." *Am J Gastroenterol.* Jan 2002;97(1):104–108.

8. Wakefield, A. J. and Montgomery, S. M. "Measles Virus as a Risk Factor for Inflammatory Bowel Disease: An Unusually Tolerant Approach." *Am J Gastroenterol.* 2000; 95:1389–1392.

9. Finn, R. "Food Allergy-Fact or Fiction: A Review." *J R Soc Med.* Sep 1992; 85(9):560–564.

10. Marteau, P. R. "Probiotics in Clinical Conditions." *Clin Rev Allergy Immunol.* Jun 2002; 22(3):255–273.

11. Fooks, L. J. and Gibson, G. R. "Probiotics as Modulators of the Gut Flora." *Br J Nutr.* Sep 2002;88 (Suppl 1):S39–49.

12. Correo, G., et al. "Mortality in Patients with Coeliac Disease and Their Relatives: A Cohort Study." *Lancet,* Aug 4, 2001;358:356–361.

13. Correo, G., et al.

14. Hodgson, H. J., et al. "Atopic Disorders and Adult Coeliac Disease." *Lancet.* Jan 17, 1976; 1(7951):115–117.

15. *MCW Health News.* December 26, 2001.

16. Carinini and Brostroff, J. "Gut and Joint Disease?" *Annals of Allergy.* 1985; 55:624–625.

17. Mainardi, E., et al. "Thyroid-related Autoantibodies and Celiac Disease: A Role for a Gluten-free Diet?" *J Clin Gastroenterol.* Sep 2002;35(3):245–248.

18. Shaul, S. A. "Gluten Intolerance: A Paradigm of an Epidemic." *Townsend Letter for Doctors & Patients.* Dec 2002;233;80–84.

19. Hoggan, R. and Braly, J. "How Modern Eating Habits May Contribute to Depression." http://depression about.com/library/weekly/aa071299.htm.

20. *Neurology.* Feb 2001;56:385–388.

21. Michaelsson, G., et al. "Psoriasis Patients with Antibodies to Gliadin Can Be Improved by a Gluten-free Diet." *British Journal of Dermatology.* 2000;142(1): 44–51.

22. Valentino, R., et al. "Markers of Potential Coeliac Disease in Patients with Hashimoto's Thyroiditis." *Eur J Endocrinol.* Apr 2002;146(4):479–483.

23. Cash, B. D., et al. "The Utility of Diagnostic Tests in Irritable Bowel Syndrome Patients: A Systematic Review." *Am J Gastroenterol.* Nov 2002;97(11): 2812–2819.

24. D'Adamo, P. and Whitney, C. *Eat Right for Your Blood Type.* (New York: Putnam Pub Group, 1996).

25. Fasano, A."Prevalence of Celiac Disease in At-risk and Not-at-risk Groups in the United States: a Large Multicenter Study." *Arch Intern Med.* Feb 10, 2003; 163(3):286–292.

Kidney Disease

1. Howanietz, H. and Lubec, G. "Idiopathic Nephrotic Syndrome, Treated with Steroids for Five Years, Found to Be Allergic Reactions to Pork." *Lancet.* Aug. 24, 1985;2(8452):450.

2. Sandberg, D. H., et al. "Severe Steroid-responsive Nephrosis Associated with Hypersensitivity." *Lancet.* Feb 19, 1977;1(8008):388–391.

Lagrue, G., et al. "Food Allergy in Idiopathic Nephrotic Syndrome." *Kidney Int Suppl.* Nov 1989;27(S):147–51.

Laurent, J., et al. "Is Adult Idiopathic Nephrotic Syndrome Food Allergy? Value of Oligoantigenic Diets." *Nephron.* 1987;47:7–11.

3. Kay, R. A. and Ferguson, A. "Intestinal T Cells, Mucosal Cell-mediated Immunity and Their Relevance to Food Allergy Disease." *Clinical Review of Allergy.* Feb 1984;2(1):56–68.

4. Sandberg, D. H.

5. Gaboardi, F., et al. "Dermatitis Herpetiformis and Nephrotic Syndrome." *Clin Nephrol.* 1983;20:49–51.

6. Selvaraj, N. "An Evaluation of Level of Oxidative Stress and Protein Glycation in Nondiabetic Undialyzed Chronic Renal Failure Patients." *Clin Chim Acta.* Oct 2002;324(1–2):45–50.

Obesity

1. Weintraub, J. M. "A Prospective Study of the Relationship Between Body Mass Index and Cataract Extraction among U.S. Women and Men." *Int J Obes Relat Metab Disord.* Dec 2002;26(12):1588–1595.

2. Gelber, A. C. "Obesity and Hip Osteoarthritis: the Weight of the Evidence Is Increasing." *Am J Med.* Feb 1, 2003;114(2):158–159.

3. "Obesity and Periodontal Disease." *J Am Dent Assoc.* Jun 15, 2000;131(6):729.

4. Heller, R. F. "Hyperinsulinemic Obesity and Carbohydrate Addiction: The Missing Link Is the Carbohydrate Frequency Factor." *Med Hypotheses.* May 1994;42(5):307–312.

5. Abbott, R. D., et al. "Midlife Adiposity and the Future Risk of Parkinson's Disease." *Neurology.* Oct 8, 2002;59(7):1051–1057.

6. BioMedNet Conference Reporter from Federation of American Societies for Experimental Biology, 1999.

7. *Ibid.*

8. Tracy, R. P. "Inflammation in Cardiovascular Disease: Cart, Horse, or Both?" *Circulation.* May 26, 2000; 97.

9. Visser, M., et al. "Low-grade Systemic Inflammation in Overweight Children." *Pediatrics.* Jan 2001;1(e13):107.

10. Lemieux, I., et al. "Elevated C-reactive Protein: Another Component of the Atherothrombotic Profile of Abdominal Obesity." *Arterioscler Thromb Vasc Biol.* 2001;21:961–067.

11. Chambers, J. C. "C-reactive Protein, Insulin Resistance, Central Obesity, and Coronary Heart Disease Risk in Indian Asians from the United Kingdom Compared with European Whites." *Circulation.* 2001;104:145–150.

12. "Obesity and Cancer." National Cancer Institute, Sept 25, 2001. http://cancer.gov/newscenter.

13. www.gsdl.com/news/connections/vol13/conn20010815.html.

Parkinson's Disease

1. Stephenson, J. "Exposure to Home Pesticides Linked to Parkinson Disease." *JAMA.* Jun 21, 2000; 283(23):3055–3056.

2. Liu, B. "Parkinson S Disease and Exposure to Infectious Agents and Pesticides and the Occurrence of Brain Injuries: Role of Neuroinflammation." *Environ Health Perspect.* 2003 Jun;111(8):1065–73.

3. Jenner, P. "Oxidative Stress in Parkinson's Disease." *Annals of Neurology.* 2003;53 Suppl 3:S26–36; discussion S36–8.

4. Ackley, D. C. and Yokel, R. A. "Aluminum Citrate Is Transported from Brain

into Blood via the Monocarboxylic Acid Transporter Located at the Blood-brain Barrier." *Toxicology.* June 27, 1997;120(2):89–97.

5. Banks, W. A. "Aluminum and Blood Brain Barrier." www.bio.unipd.it/ ~zatta/ banks.htm.

6. Metals—International Occupational Safety and Health Information Centre, 1999. www.ilo.org/public/english/protection/safework/cis/products/safe-tytm/metals.htm.

7. "Parkinson's Disease Linked To High Iron Intake." www.sciencedaily.com/ releases/2003/06/030610081311.htm.

8. Pall, H. S., et al. "Raised Cerebrospinal-fluid Copper Concentration in Parkinson's Disease." *Lancet.* Aug 1,1987; 2(8553):238–241.

9. Pellecchia, M. T. "Possible Gluten Sensitivity in Multiple System Atrophy." *Neurology.* Oct 8, 2002; 59(7):1114–5.

10. Carratu, P., et al. "Evaluation of Leakage of Bacteria and Endotoxins in Teeth Treated Endodontically by Two Different Techniques." *J Endod.* Apr 2002; 28(4):272–5.

11. Shefrin, S. L. "Therapeutic Advances in Idiopathic Parkinsonism." *Expert Opin Investig Drugs.* Oct 1999; (10):1565–1588.

12. "Excitotoxins, Neurodegeneration and Neurodevelopment." Blaylock, M. D. www.dorway.com/blayenn.html.

13. Czlonkowska, A., et al. "Immune Processes in the Pathogenesis of Parkinson's Disease—a Potential Role for Microglia and Nitric Oxide." *Med Sci Monit.* 2002 Aug;8(8):RA165–77.

14. Hellenbrand, W. "Diet and Parkinson's Disease. A Possible Role for the Past Intake of Specific Nutrients. Results from a Self-administered Food-frequency Questionnaire in a Case-control Study." *Neurology.* Sep 1996;47(3):644–650.

15. Logroscino, G., et al. "Dietary Lipids and Antioxidants in Parkinson's Disease: a Population-based, Case-control Study." *Ann Neurol.* Jan 1996; 39(1):89–94.

Periodontal Disease

1. LeResche, L. and Dworkin, S. F. "The Role of Stress in Inflammatory Disease, Including Periodontal Disease: Review of Concepts and Current Findings." *Periodontol.* 2002; 30:91–103.

2. Teng, Y. T., et al. "Periodontal Health and Systemic Disorders." *J Can Dent Assoc.* Mar 2002; 68(3): 188–192.

3. Chapple, I. L. "Glutathione in Gingival Crevicular Fluid and Its Relation to Local Antioxidant Capacity in Periodontal Health and Disease." *Mol Pathol.* Dec 2002; 55(6):367–373.

4. Hildebrand, H. C., et al. "The Influence of Psychological Stress on Periodontal Disease." *J West Soc Periodontol Periodontal.* 2000; 48(3):69–77.

5. Reed, B. E., et al. "Orofacial Sensitivity Reactions and the Role of Dietary Components. Case Reports." *Aust Dent J.* Aug 1993;38(4):287–291.

6. Geerts, S.O., et al. "Systemic Release of Endotoxins Induced by Gentle Masti-

cation: Association with Periodontitis Severity." *Journal of Periodontology.* Jan 2002;73:73–78.

7. Tomar, S. L. and Asthma, S. "Smoking-attributable Periodontitis in the United States: Findings from Nhanes Iii." *J Periodontol.* 2000;71:743–751.

8. LeResche, L. and Dworkin, S. F. "The Role of Stress in Inflammatory Disease, Including Periodontal Disease: Review of Concepts and Current Findings." *J Can Dent Assoc.* Mar 2002;68(3):188–192.

9. Singer, R. E., et al. "Relationship between Gingivital Inflammation and Systemic Bio-Markers:Impact of Smoking and Systemic Anti-Oxidants." *P & G Dental Resource.* www.dentalcare.com/soap/journals/pgresrch/posters/ iadr02/pp 802.htm.

10. Lappin, D. F. "Inducible Nitric Oxide Synthase Expression in Periodontitis." *J Periodontal Res.* Dec 2000; 35(6):369–373.

Pregnancy, Infancy and Childhood Problems

1. Ozanne, S. H. "Early Programming of Glucose-Insulin Metabolism." *Trends Endocrinol Metab.* Nov 13, 2002;9:368.

2. Pressinger, R. W. "Learning Disability Research." www.chem-tox.com/ pregnancy/learning_disabilities.htm.

3. Wilson, W. H. "Recurrent Acute Otitis Media in Infants—Role of Immune Complexes Acquired in Utero." *Laryngoscope.* Apr 1983;93(4): 418–421.

4. Offenbacher, S., et al. "Periodontal Infection as a Possible Risk Factor for Preterm Low Birth Weight." *Journal of Periodontology.* 1996; 67(10 suppl): 1103–1113.

5. Marini, A., et al. "Effects of a Dietary and Environmental Prevention Programme on the Incidence of Allergic Symptoms in High Atopic Risk Infants: Three Years' Follow-up." *Acta Paed Suppl.* 1996; 414:1–21.

6. Ulett, G. "Food Allergy-Cytotoxic Testing and the Central Nervous System." *Psychiatric Journal of the University of Ottawa.* 8:2: June 1, 1980, 100–108.

7. Heiner, D. C. "Respiratory Disease and Food Allergy." *Ann Allergy.* Dec 1984; 53:657–664.

8. Morris, I. G. "Gamma Globulin Absorption in the Newborn in C.F." Cope, ed. *Handbook of Physiology of the Alimentary Canal,* Vol.2, (Washington, DC: American Physiological Society, 1968)1491–1512.

9. Mathew, D. J., et al. "Prevention of Eczema." *Lancet.* Feb 12, 1977;1(8007): 321–324.

10. Lucarelli, S., et al. "Food Allergy and Infantile Autism." *Panminerva Medica.* Sep 1995;37(3):137–141.

11. Businco, I. "Chronic Diarrhea Due to Cow's Milk Allergy, A 4 to 10 Year Follow-op Study." *Annals of Allergy.* Dec 1985:55, 844–847.

12. D'Eufemia, P., et al. "Abnormal Intestinal Permeability in Children with Autism." *Acta Paediatrica.* Sep 1996; 85(9):1076–1079.

13. Wakefield, A. J., et al. "Enterocolitis in Children With Developmental Disorders." *American Journal of Gastroenterology.* Sept 2000; 95:2285–2295.

14. Bellanti, J. A. 59th Annual Meeting of the American College of Allergy, Asthma, and Immunology.

15. Rapp, D. J. "Does Diet Affect Hyperactivity?" *J Learning Dis.* 1978; 11:383–389.

Boris, M. and Mandel, F. S. "Foods and Additives Are Common Causes of the Attention Deficit Hyperactive Disorder in Children." *Ann Allergy.* 1994; 72:462–468.

16. Heyman, M., et al. "Mononuclear Cells from Infants Allergic to Cow's Milk Secrete Tumor Necrosis Factor Alpha, Altering Intestinal Function." *Gastroenterology.* Jun 1994; 106(6): 1514–1523.

17. Huynh, H. K. and Dorovinizis, K. "Effects of Interferon-gamma on Primary Cultures of Human Brain Microvessel Endothelial Cells." *Am Jour Path.* Apr 1993; 142(4): 1265–1278.

18. Uhlmann, V., et al. "Potential Viral Pathogenic Mechanism for New Variant Inflammatory Bowel Disease." *Mol Pathol.* Apr 2002; 55(2): 84–90.

19. Panksepp, J. "Neurohumoral and Endocrine Control of Feeding." *Psychoneuroendocrinology.* 1979; 4(2): 89–106.

Respiratory Disease

1. Heiner, D. C. "Respiratory Diseases and Food Allergy." *Ann Allergy.* Dec 1984; 53:657–664.

2. *Ibid.*

3. Rowe, A. H., et al., "Food Allergy–Its Role in the Symptoms of Obstructive Emphysema and Chronic Bronchitis." *J Asthma Res.* Sep 1967;5(1):11–20.

4. Freedman, B. J. "Asthma Induced by Sulphur Dioxide, Benzoate and Tartrazine Contained in Orange Drinks." *Clin Allergy.* 1977; 7:407–415.

5. Marwick, J. A. et al. "Cigarette Smoke-induced Oxidative Stress and Tgf-beta1 Increase P21waf1/cip1 Expression in Alveolar Epithelial Cells." *Ann N Y Acad Sci.* Nov. 2002; 973:278–283.

6. Peroni, D. G., et al. "Food Allergy: What Can Be Done to Prevent Progression to Asthma?" *Ann Allergy Asthma Immunol.* Dec 2002;89(6 Suppl 1):44–51.

7. Agusti, A.G.N., et al. "Systemic Effects of Chronic Obstructive Pulmonary Disease." *Euro Res J.* 21(2):347–360.

Rheumatic Diseases

1. Solomon, D. H., et al. "Cardiovascular Morbidity and Mortality in Women Diagnosed with Rheumatoid Arthritis." *Circulation.* Feb 2003; 10.1161–1201.

2. Hurlimann, D. "Anti-tumor Necrosis Factor-alpha Treatment Improves Endothelial Function in Patients with Rheumatoid Arthritis." *Circulation.* Oct 22, 2002; 106(17): 2184–2187.

3. Darlington, L.G. "Placebo-Controlled, Blind Study of Dietary Manipulation Therapy in Rheumatoid Arthritis." *Lancet.* Feb. 6, 1986; 236–238.

Cleland, L.G. "Diet and Arthritis." *Bailieres Clin Rheumatol.* Nov. 1995; 9(4): 771–785.

Catteral, W.E. "Rheumatoid Arthritis Is an Allergy." *Arthritis News Today.* 1980.

4. Carinini, C. and Brostroff, J. "Gut and Joint Disease." *Annals of Allergy.* 1985; 55:624–625.

5. Little, C., et al. "Platelet Serotonin Release in Rheumatoid Arthritis: A Study in Food Intolerant Patients." *Lancet.* Aug 6,1983;2(8345)297–299.

6. Parke, A., et al. "Celiac Disease and Rheumatoid Arthritis." *Annals of Rheum Dis.* 1984, 43:378–380.

7. American College of Rheumatology's Annual Meeting, San Francisco. November 13, 2001.

8. Ratner, D. "Juvenile Rheumatoid Arthritis and Milk Allergy." *J R Soc Med.* 1985; 78:410–413.

Ratner, D., et al."Does Milk Intolerance Affect Seronegative Arthritis in Lactase-deficient Women? *Isr J Med Sci.* 1985;21:532–534.

9. Beri, D., et al. "Effect of Dietary Restrictions on Disease Activity in Rheumatoid Arthritis." *Ann Rheum Dis.* 1988;47:69–72.

10. "Allergy Health." http://homedoctor.net/tipsfaq/1.5.html.

11. Ratner, D. "Juvenile Rheumatoid Arthritis and Milk Allergy." *JR Soc Med.* May 1985(5);410–3.

12. Katz, J. P. and Lichtenstein, G. R. "Rheumatologic Manifestations of Gastrointestinal Diseases" *Gastroenterol Clin North Am.* Sep 1998;27(3):533–62.

13. Gislason, S. J. "Chemical Sensitivities." www.nutramed.com/environment/mcs.htm.

14. Krohn, K. "Symptoms of Fibromyalgia." www.coloradohealthsite.org/fibro/fibro_oregon.html.

15. *Ibid.*

16. Brown, A. C. "Lupus Erythematosus and Nutrition." *J Ren Nutr* Oct 10, 2000;4:170–183

17. *Ibid.*

18. Machtelincks, V. "Lupus Erythematosus and Allergy." www.cibliga.com/en/a_m_sle_allergie.html.

19. Childers, N. F. "A Relationship of Arthritis to the Solanaceae (Nightshades)." *J Inernat Ac Pre.* Nov 1982:31–37.

20. Zautra, A. J., et al. "Field Research on the Relationship Between Stress and Disease Activity in Rheumatoid Arthritis." *Ann NY Acad Sci.* June 22, 1999; 876:397–412.

21. Potter, P. T. "Interpersonal Workplace Stressors and Well-being: a Multi-wave Study of Employees with and Without Arthritis." *J Appl Psychol.* Aug 2002;87(4):789–796.

22. Hauschildt, E. "Glycation Levels Could Affect Progression of Osteoarthritis." http://www3.interscience.wiley.com/cgi-bin/abstract/88010819/ START.

23. Drinda, S., et al. "Identification of the Advanced Glycation End Products N-carboxymethyllysine in the Synovial Tissue of Patients with Rheumatoid Arthritis." *Ann Rheum Dis*. 2002;61:488–492.

Surgery Problems

1. Udelsman, R. and Holbrook, N. J. "Endocrine and Molecular Responses to Surgical Stress." *Curr Probl Surg*. Aug 1994;31(8):653–720.

2. Salo, M., et al. "Effects of Anaesthesia and Surgery on the Immune Response." *Acta Anaesthesiol Scand*. Apr 1992;36(3):201–220.

3. *Ibid*.

4. Schots, R. "Monitoring of C-reactive Protein after Allogeneic Bone Marrow Transplantation Identifies Patients at Risk of Severe Transplant-related Complications and Mortality." *Bone Marrow Transplant*. Jul 1998;22(1):79–85.

5. Phan, T. G., et al. *Archives of Internal Medicine*. Jan 27, 2003;163:237–239.

Conclusion

1. Matteo, A. and Sarles, H. "Is Food Allergy a Cause of Acute Pancreatitis?" *Pancreas*. Mar 1990;5(2):234–237.

2. Ames, B. N., et al. "Oxidants, Antioxidants, and the Degenerative Diseases of Aging." *Proc Natl Acad Sci* (USA) 1993;90:7915–7920.

3. De Muro, P., and Ficari, A. "Experimental Studies on Allergic Cholecystitis." *Gastroenterology*. 1946;6:302–314.

4. Collin, P. "Celiac Disease in Patients with Severe Liver Disease: Gluten-free Diet May Reverse Hepatic Failure." *Gastroenterology*. 2002;122:881–888.

5. Wright, J. "Premenstrual Syndrome." www.healthy.net/library/Audio/Wright/problems/pms.htm.

Chapter 6

1. Kushner, I. "Semantics, Inflammation, Cytokines and Common Sense." *Cytokine Growth Factor Rev*. 1998; 9:191_196.

Chapter 7

1. Montalto, M., et al. "Probiotics: History, Definition, Requirements and Possible Therapeutic Applications." *Ann Ital Med Int*. Jul-Sep 2002;17(3):157–165.

2. Simopoulos, A. P. "Omega-3 Fatty Acids in Inflammation and Autoimmune Diseases." *J Am Coll Nutr*. Dec 2002;21(6):495–505.

3. Ford, E. "Does Exercise Reduce Inflammation? Physical Activity and C-reactive Protein among Us Adults." *Epidemiology*. 2002;13:561–568 .

4. Suzuki, K., et al. "Endurance Exercise Causes Interaction among Stress Hormones, Cytokines, Neutrophil Dynamics and Muscle Damage." *J Appl Physiol*. 1999; 87:13601367.

5. de Maat, M. P. and Kluft, C. "The Association Between Inflammation Markers, Coronary Artery Disease and Smoking." *Vascul Pharmacol.* Aug 2002;39(3): 137–139.

6. Agusti, A. G. "Systemic Effects of Chronic Obstructive Pulmonary Disease." *Eur Respir J.* Feb 2003;21(2):347–360.

7. "Secondhand Smoke Exposure Among Middle and High School Students–Texas, 2001." *MMWR Morb Mortal Wkly Rep.* Feb 28, 2003;52(8): 152–154.

8. Philip Morris USA. www.pmusa.com/health_issues/cigarette_smoking_and _disease.asp.

9. Reynold, K. "Alcohol Consumption and Risk of Stroke." *JAMA.* 2003;289: 579–580.

10. Davis, J."Booze Could Be Tied to Allergy Blues." WebMD Medical News.

11. Winger, "Conquering Alcoholic Liver Disease." *Medical Alumni Bulletin.* UCN School of Medicine, 1995/1996.

12. "The Alternative Advisor: The Complete Guide to Natural Therapies and Alternative Treatments—Time-Life Books 1997." The 1997—1998 Special Edition of *New Age Journal.*

13. "Causes of Sinusitis." Seniorhealth.about.com.

14. Miller, G. E. "Chronic Psychological Stress and the Regulation of Pro-inflammatory Cytokines: A Glucocorticoid-resistance Model." *Health Psychol.* Nov 2002;21(6):531–541.

15. *Ibid.*

16. Spiegel, K., et al. "Impact of Sleep Debt on Metabolic and Endocrine Function." *Lancet.* Oct 23, 1999; 354:1435_1439.

17. Mercola, J. with Levy, A. R. *The No-Grain Diet.* (New York: Dutton, 2003).

18. *Clinical Chemistry* 2002; 48:877.

Chapter 8

1. Helke, F. "Detoxify—Buzzword of a New Era." *Vitality Magazine.* Nov 2002:6.

2. D'Adamo, P. J. and Whitney, C. (Contributor). *Eat Right for Your Blood Type.* (New York:Putnam Publishing Group, 1996).

3. Fedorak, R. N., and Madsen, K. L. "Probiotics and Prebiotics in Gastrointestinal Disorders." *Curr Opin Gastroenterol* 20(2):146–155, 2004.

4. Ferrie, H. "New Perspectives in the War on Cancer." *Vitality Magazine,* Fall 1999, Toronto, Canada.

About the Author

Nancy Appleton earned her BS in clinical nutrition from UCLA and her PhD in health services from Walden University. She maintains a private practice in Santa Monica, California. An avid researcher, Dr. Appleton lecturers extensively throughout the world, and has appeared on numerous television and radio talk shows. Her main interest is homeostasis, balance in the body, what causes the body to lose its delicate balance, and what we can do to regain and maintain homeostasis. She is the best-selling author of *Lick the Sugar Habit*, *Lick the Sugar Habit Counter*, *Healthy Bones*, *Heal Yourself with Natural Foods*, and *Rethinking Louis Pasteur's Germ Theory*. She currently lives in Santa Monica, California.

Index

Order Forms

AUDIO CASSETTES

Lick the Sugar Habit—An introduction to the book, this tape provides detailed explanations of the body chemistry princlple, mineral relationships, the endocrine system, enzymes, and promoters of infectious and degenerative disease. (1 hour)

Allergies—What are food allergies? What causes them to come? How can they be eliminated? Learn how foods to which you have an a allergic reaction can be reintroduced in your diet. Environmental allergies are also discussed. (1 hour)

Osteoporosis—Although you may be getting a reasonable amount of calcium in your diet, if your body chemistry is upset, the calcium cannot be absorbed properly. Thsi tape explains how to look for symptoms of calcium deficiency and how to test for susceptibility to osteoporosis. (1 hour)

Obesity—The latest research on the relationship of allergies, addictions, and cravings to obesity is presented. (30 minutes) **Women** is on flip side of the tape.

Women—Information on premenstrual syndrome (PMS), candidiasis (yeast infections), menstruation, menopause, and postmenopausal problems is presented. (30 minutes) **Obesity** is on the flip side.

Children—This tape begins with a discussion of prenatal nutrition. Information on food allergies and eating problems for infants and children follows. Ideas for encouraging older children and teenagers to eat nutritious foods end the tape. (1 hour)

Food Preparation—This tape answers the following questions. Where can I shop for the most nutritious foods? How can I prepare food to keep it from upsetting my body's delicate chemical balance? What I should know about food additives, irradiation, insecticides, and fungicides? (1 hour)

Urine and pH Testing—Information and instruction for testing homeostasis through saliva and urine are presented. Common causes of upset body chemistry are discussed, as well as ways to regain the body's chemical balance. (1 hour)

How Our Diet Affects Our Immune System—Lecture Dr. Appleton gave concerning how our diet can either enhance our immune system or exhaust our immune system opening the door to infectious and degenerative diseases. ($1\frac{1}{2}$ hours)

Audio Cassette Order Form

Name _____

Address _____ Apt _____

City _____ State _____ Zip _____

List Cassette titles:

1.   5.

2.   6.

3.   7.

4.   8.

PRICE LIST			
QUANTITY	PRICE (US CURRENCY)	SHIPPING	SHIPPING TO CANADA
1	$ 7.00	$ 1.50	$ 1.75
2	$12.00	$ 1.75	$ 2.00
3	$15.00	$ 2.00	$ 2.25
4	$20.00	$ 2.25	$ 2.50
5	$25.00	$ 2.50	$ 2.75
6	$30.00	$ 2.75	$ 3.00
7	$35.00	$ 3.00	$ 3.25
8	$40.00	$ 3.25	$ 3.50 .

* California residents, please apply appropriate sales tax or 10%.

Mail this completed form along with a chek made payable to Nancy Appleton, PhD to:

Nancy Appleton, PhD
P.O. Box 3083
Santa Monica, CA 90403

You can also contact Nancy Appleton at info@nancyappleton.com or visit her website at www.nancyappleton.com.

BODY CHEMISTRY TEST KIT

The kit contains tests that determine if your body chemistry is in homeostasis, in balance. Solutions for 250 tests, two test tubes, an eye-dropper, a brush for cleaning the test tubes, and pH paper for testing the acid/alkalinity of the urine and saliva are included. An informative twenty-eight page booklet, *Monitoring Your Basic Health*, contains information on body chemistry, what upsets it, how to regain and maintain it. The booklet also provides suggested food plans and instructions on how to test for food allergies. The two accompanying audiocassette tapes, "How Our Diet Affects Our Immune System (1½ hours) and "pH and Urine Testing (1 hour), will give you a further understanding of homeostasis and of the testing process.

Body Chemistry Test Kit Order Form

Name _____

Address _____ Apt _____

City _____ State _____ Zip _____

Cost of Body Chemistry Test Kit

1 Kit	$30.00
Shipping	$ 3.50
Shipping to Canada (US currency)	$ 4.50
California residents*	$
TOTAL	$

*California residents please add appropriate sales tax or 10%

Mail this completed form along with a chek made payable to Nancy Appleton, PhD to:

Nancy Appleton, PhD
P.O. Box 3083
Santa Monica, CA 90403

You can also contact Nancy Appleton at info@nancyappleton.com or visit her website at www.nancyappleton.com.

OTHER SQUAREONE TITLES OF INTEREST

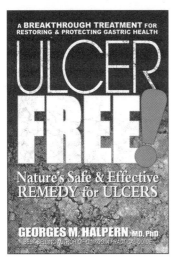

A BREAKTHROUGH TREATMENT FOR RESTORING & PROTECTING GASTRIC HEALTH

ULCER FREE!
Nature's Safe and Effective Remedy for Ulcers
Georges M. Halpern, MD

Over 4 million Americans are diagnosed annually with peptic ulcer disease. Many learn to live with the resulting heartburn, acid reflux, nausea, gas, and stomach pain with the help of over-the-counter antacids. These products may stop the pain, but only temporarily. Furthermore, the underlying condition can worsen. But it doesn't have to be that way. *Ulcer Free!* is a practical guide to understanding the causes of and effective treatments for peptic ulcer disease.

The book begins with a look at why we get ulcers. It examines the *Helicobacter pylori* bacterium—the culprit behind the majority of stomach ulcers. It also discusses the growing number of ulcers caused by NSAIDs—over-the-counter pain relievers, more commonly known as aspirin, ibuprofen, naproxen, and a variety of other products. The book then offers an unbiased look at the treatments--conventional and alternative--that can stop the symptoms of and actually heal ulcers. Finally, *Ulcer Free!* introduces the breakthrough nutrient Zinc-Carnosine, which can be used in conjunction with other treatments or on its own.

If you are tired of being victim to continual gastric distress, *Ulcer Free!* can help. Up-to-date and accurate, it offers the key to permanent relief.

Georges M. Halpern, MD, attended medical school at the University of Paris, France. He subsequently received a PhD from the Faculty of Pharmacy, University of Paris XI—Chatenay Malabry. A Fellow of the American Academy of Allergy and Immunology, Dr. Halpern is board certified in internal medicine and allergy, and is Professor Emeritus of Medicine at the University of California—Davis. He is also a Distinguished Professor of Medicine at the University of Hong Kong.

AVAILABLE $14.95 US / $22.50 CAN • 208 pages • 6 x 9-inch quality paperback
Health/Ulcers • ISBN 0-7570-0253-6

THE MAGNESIUM SOLUTION FOR HIGH BLOOD PRESSURE
How to Use Magnesium to Help Prevent and Relieve Hypertension Naturally
Jay S. Cohen, MD

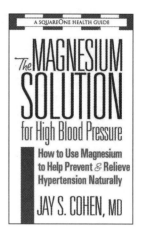

Approximately 50 percent of all Americans have hypertension, a devastating disease that can lead to hardening of the arteries, heart attack, and stroke. While many medications are available to combat this condition, these drugs come with potentially dangerous side effects. When Dr. Jay S. Cohen learned of his own vascular condition, he was well aware of the risks associated with standard treatments. Based upon his research, he selected a safer option—magnesium.

In *The Magnesium Solution for High Blood Pressure,* Dr. Cohen describes the most effective types of magnesium for treating hypertension, explores appropriate magnesium dosage, and details the use of magnesium in conjunction with hypertension meds. Here is a proven remedy for anyone looking for a safe, effective approach to the treatment of high blood pressure.

$5.95 • 96 pages • 4 x 7.5-inch mass paperback • Health/High Blood Pressure • ISBN 0-7570-0255-2

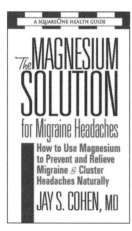

THE MAGNESIUM SOLUTION FOR MIGRAINE HEADACHES
How to Use Magnesium to Prevent and Relieve Migraine and Cluster Headaches Naturally
Jay S. Cohen, MD

More than 30 million people across North America suffer from migraine headaches. Over the years, a number of drugs have been developed to treat migraines, but these treatments don't work for everyone, and come with a high risk of side effects. Fortunately, Dr. Jay S. Cohen has discovered an alternative—magnesium.

This easy-to-understand guide explains what a migraine is, and shows how this supplement can play a key role in preventing and treating migraine headaches. It also describes what type of magnesium works best, and how much magnesium should be taken to prevent or stop migraines. For those who are looking for a safe and effective approach to the prevention and treatment of migraine and cluster headaches, Dr. Cohen prescribes a proven natural remedy in *The Magnesium Solution for Migraine Headaches.*

$5.95 • 96 pages • 4 x 7.5-inch mass paperback • Health/Migraines • ISBN 0-7570-0256-0

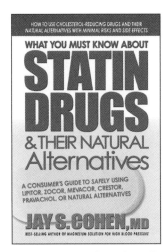

What You Must Know About Statin Drugs & Their Natural Alternatives

A Consumer's Guide to Safely Using Lipitor, Zocor, Mevacor, Crestor, Pravachol, or Natural Alternatives

Jay S. Cohen, MD

It is estimated that over 100 million Americans suffer from elevated cholesterol and C-reactive proteins—markers that are linked to heart attack, stroke, and other cardiovascular disorders. To combat these problems, modern science has created a group of drugs known either as statins or as specific commercial drugs such as Lipitor, Zocor, and Pravachol. While over 20 million people take these medications, the fact is that up to 42 percent experience side effects, and a whopping 60 to 70 percent eventually stop treatment. Here, for the first time, is a guide that explains the problems caused by statins, and offers easy-to-follow strategies that will allow you to benefit from these drugs while avoiding their side effects. In addition, the author provides natural alternatives that have also proven effective.

What You Must Know About Statin Drugs & Their Natural Alternatives begins by explaining elevated cholesterol and C-reactive proteins. It then examines how statins work to alleviate these problems, and discusses possible side effects. Highlighted is information on safe usage, as well as a discussion of effective alternative treatments. If you have elevated cholesterol and C-reactive proteins, or if you are currently using a statin, *What You Must Know About Statin Drugs & Their Natural Alternatives* can make a profound difference in the quality of your life.

Jay S. Cohen, MD, an Associate Professor (voluntary) of Family and Preventive Medicine at the University of California, San Diego, found relief from a disabling vascular disorder with magnesium. Dr. Cohen is a widely recognized expert on prescription drugs and their natural alternatives. He has published scientific papers in leading medical journals and has written articles for *Newsweek, Bottom Line Health*, and *Life Extension Magazine*. Dr. Cohen is a highly sought-after speaker and publishes commentary for the public on current issues in health care at www.MedicationSense.com. Dr. Cohen practices preventive and integrative medicine in Del Mar, California.

$15.95 • 204 pages • 6 x 9-inch paperback • Health • ISBN 0-7570-0257-9

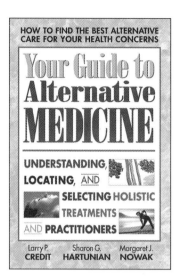

HOW TO FIND THE BEST ALTERNATIVE CARE FOR YOUR HEALTH CONCERNS

Your Guide to Alternative MEDICINE

UNDERSTANDING, LOCATING, AND SELECTING HOLISTIC TREATMENTS AND PRACTITIONERS

Larry P. CREDIT   Sharon G. HARTUNIAN   Margaret J. NOWAK

YOUR GUIDE TO ALTERNATIVE MEDICINE

Understanding, Locating, and Selecting Holistic Treatments and Practitioners

Larry P. Credit, Sharon G. Hartunian, and Margaret J. Nowak

The growing world of complementary medicine offers safe and effective solutions to many health disorders, from backache to headache. You may already be interested in alternative care approaches, but if you're like most people, you have a hundred and one questions you'd like answered before you choose a treatment. "Will I feel the acupuncture needles?" "What is a homeopathic remedy?" "Does chiropractic hurt?" *Your Guide to Alternative Medicine* provides the fundamental facts necessary to choose an effective complementary care therapy and begin treatment.

This comprehensive reference clearly explains numerous approaches in an easy-to-read format. For every complementary care option discussed, there is a description and brief history; a list of conditions that respond; information on the cost and duration of treatment; credentials and educational background for practitioners; and more. To find those therapies most appropriate for a specific condition, there is even a unique troubleshooting chart.

Your Guide to Alternative Medicine introduces you to options that you may never have considered—techniques that enhance the body's natural healing potential and have few, if any, side effects. Here is a reference that can help you make informed decisions about all your important healthcare needs.

$11.95 • 208 pages • 6 x 9-inch quality paperback • Health/Alternative Therapies/Reference ISBN 0-7570-0125-4

For more information about our books, visit our website at www.squareonepublishers.com